the detox plan

for body, mind, and spirit

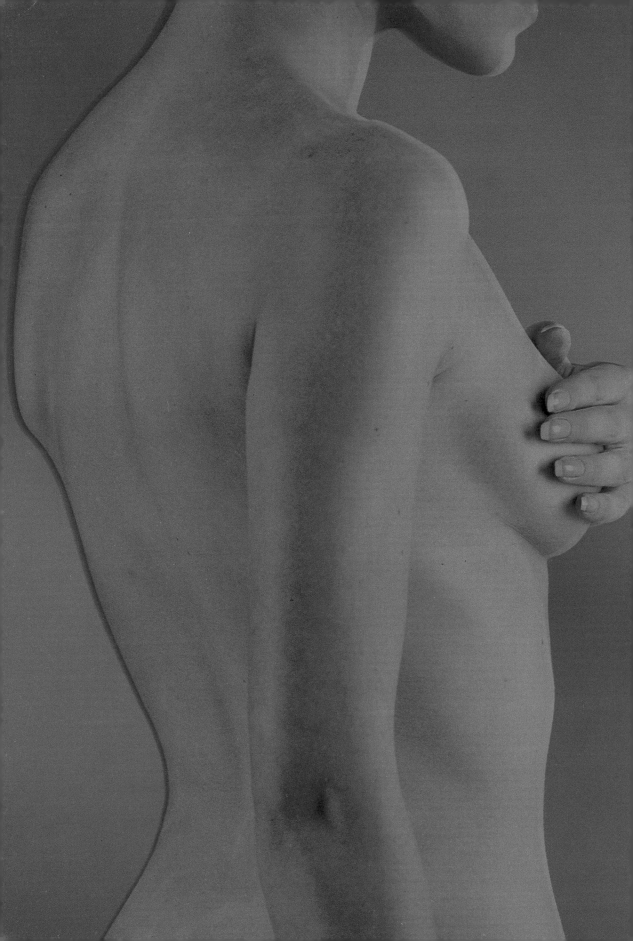

the detox plan

for body, mind, and spirit

Jane Alexander

JOURNEY EDITIONS
BOSTON • TOKYO

First published in the United States in 1998 by Journey Editions, an imprint of Periplus Editions (HK) Ltd., with editorial offices at 153 Milk Street, Boston, Massachusetts 02109.

DISCLAIMER

The author of this book is not a physician, and the ideas, procedures, and suggestions in this book are intended to supplement, not replace, the medical and legal advice of trained professionals.

All matters regarding your health require medical supervision. Consult your medical practitioner before adopting the suggestions in this book, as well as about any condition that may require diagnosis or medical attention.

The author and publisher of this book are not responsible in any manner whatsoever for any injury that may occur directly or indirectly from use of this book.

ISBN: 1-885203-70-5

Library of Congress Catalog Card Number: 98-86035

Distributed by

USA
Charles E. Tuttle Co., Inc.
RR 1 Box 231-5
North Clarendon, VT 05759
Tel.: (802) 773-8930
Fax.: (802) 773-6993

Japan
Tuttle Shokai Ltd.
1-21-13, Seki
Tama-ku, Kawasaki-shi
Kanagawa-ken 214, Japan
Tel.: (044) 833-0225
Fax.: (044) 822-0413

Southeast Asia
Berkeley Books Pte. Ltd.
5 Little Road #08-01
Singapore 536983
Tel.: (65) 280-3320
Fax.: (65) 280-6290

First edition
05 04 03 02 01 00 99 98   10 9 8 7 6 5 4 3 2 1
Design by Phil Gamble

Printed by Printer Trento Srl, Italy

Introduction

Imagine waking up each morning full of energy and vitality yet also feeling calm and relaxed about the day to come. It sounds like a miracle yet this state of abundant health and vibrant wellbeing should be our birthright. In our natural state we would face each day with joy, peace, and a deep connection with our bodies.

So why do so many of us feel so bad? Much of it can be blamed on toxicity. Everywhere we turn we are assaulted by toxins: in the air we breathe, the food we eat, and the water we drink. Allergies and sensitivities are on the increase, many caused by the growing levels of pollution in the environment, chemicals in our homes, and additives in our food.

It is not just our bodies which bear the brunt either. Our minds are overloaded with increasing work and the deep stresses and strains of coping in a complicated world. When mind and body are assaulted, we feel physically unwell, emotionally drained, and psychically bereft.

Some people give up, thinking that since toxins are so prevalent why try to combat them? Equally, others fall into the opposite camp, living a miserable life wrapped in seaweed and permanently fasting! But there is a middle way. We can reduce our toxic overload and regain the equilibrium we all so desperately need and desire. The aim of this book is to provide a straightforward, simple, and surprisingly enjoyable guide to coping with our toxic world. We'll take a realistic look at the toxic threat, pinpointing precisely where the major problems lie, and provide clear advice about how you can reduce your own personal toxic load.

The final chapter offers a guide to your own personal detox program. You can choose either a full one-month program, which can be easily fitted into your everyday life, or decide on a weekend "retreat from the world". If you have sensitivities, allergies, or intolerances, straightforward advice can help you detect the culprits.

The book gives you the opportunity to transform your life. In an increasingly scary world, it lets you take back control over your health and wellbeing. It gives you the chance to make a clean, fresh start.

Jane Alexander

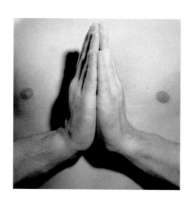

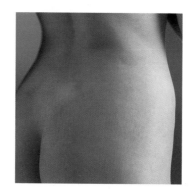

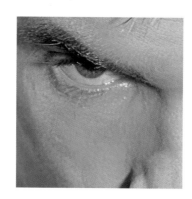

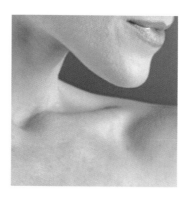

Contents

Chapter One

The good, the bad, and the toxic

The modern world is a toxic battleground. Begin the fightback to health by finding out where a whole range of toxins accumulate in your life – in your food, your home, and your workplace.

Why do we need to detox? In an ideal world our bodies would quietly detoxify without any extra help from us. After all, bodies are naturally designed to deal with a whole host of threats as part of everyday life: from bacteria and viruses to shocks and frights. The problems arise because in the modern world there is just too much for the body to cope with and so our natural systems of elimination cannot handle the strain.

And what a strain it is. Our bodies are sloughing off an incredible amount of rubbish each and every day – in our urine and stools; in sweat and the exhalation of gases. Some is metabolic waste, dead cells, the by-products of digestion, and other natural debris. But more and more of it is toxic waste: pesticides, food additives, drugs, the chemicals we inhale from pollution, and even everyday household products.

Throughout this book we will be looking at ways to encourage the vital detox mechanisms of our bodies to work at their optimum best. Let's take a swift look at the body's unique system of detoxing, in particular our liver, skin, lungs, kidneys, intestines, and lymphatic system, to get a picture of how they process and eliminate toxins. Then we'll concentrate on the importance of healthy food and a clean environment – the answers you give to the questionnaires that follow will help you discover where to start detoxing.

Don't be discouraged if you score highly in these questionnaires – you will not be alone. This is a starting point, a chance to evaluate your lifestyle and identify major problems. Ask how you can reduce obvious problems – don't change jobs or give up activities but remember, little shifts can make a huge difference.

YOUR TOXIC OVERLOAD

How toxic is your life right now? Which areas of your life are causing this toxicity? Answering these questions honestly is the first step on the road to detoxing.

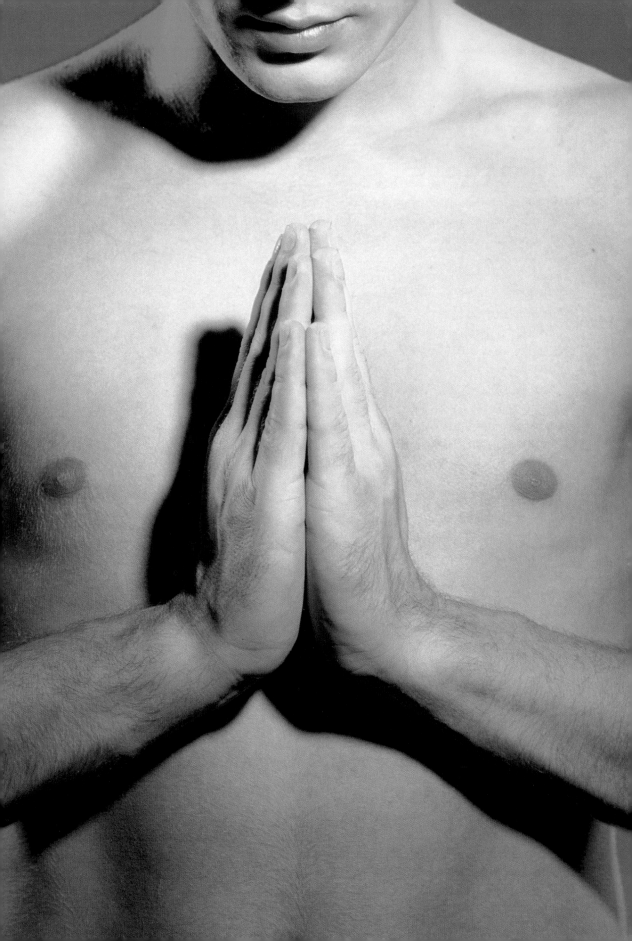

The body's own way of detoxing

Detoxing is a non-stop process. Our bodies are undergoing a constant process of cleaning out, getting rid of every molecule that has served its purpose as well as eliminating unwelcome toxins and metabolic waste. At the same time, brand new molecules are being produced to help dispose of bodily waste. The detox system is complex and, in order to help it function at its best, we need to take a holistic approach to our health. However, it's also worth knowing a little about the main players in the detox game…

The lymphatic system

This is the body's trash collection system. The lymph (a milky fluid that contains a type of white blood cell, proteins, and fat) moves slowly around the body. As it passes through one of a multitude of lymph nodes, foreign bodies or toxins are filtered out from the lymph. Infections are fought here and any poisonous material is prevented from going back into the bloodstream.

The liver

The liver has to deal with virtually everything that comes into the body, clearing the blood of poisonous substances (everything from alcohol to pesticides) that would otherwise build up in the bloodstream. It absorbs these toxins, alters their chemical structure, makes them water soluble, and then excretes them into the bile (a greenish-brown liquid). The bile then carries these waste products away from the liver to the intestines from which they are excreted.

The lungs

Millions of tiny air sacs in our lungs provide us with about 50 square metres (540 square feet) for the exchange of gases. When we breathe, oxygen enters the blood and the waste products of respiration (carbon dioxide and water) are removed. The lungs also have to cope with a host of air-borne pollutants, such as carbon monoxide from traffic fumes, nicotine from cigarette smoke, and formaldehyde from building materials and fabrics.

THE LYMPHATIC SYSTEM
This elaborate network of lymph channels filters the fluid in the body's tissues and transfers the toxins to the blood. Lymph nodes may be as large as a pea or as small as a pinhead.

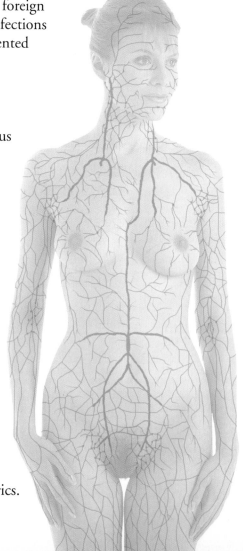

The kidneys

The prime function of the kidneys is to filter the blood and produce urine, removing toxins and waste products generated by the breakdown of proteins. They also control the body's acidity and water levels, and put back into the blood any valuable nutrients that need to be recycled for further use.

The skin

The skin is the body's largest organ – if spread out flat it would cover about 1.5 square metres (17 square feet). It is a wonderful detoxifier; its sweat and sebaceous glands remove and slough off toxins that cannot be eliminated by any other means.

The intestines

Our intestines break down and absorb food and water into the bloodstream, and carry away the waste products of digestion and liver metabolism. A well-functioning digestive system moves waste swiftly out of the body. However, a highly processed diet often leads to constipation, with toxic waste remaining in the body far longer than necessary.

SIGNS OF IMBALANCE WITHIN YOUR BODY'S DETOX SYSTEM	
The Lymphatic System	*frequent colds and flu; tiredness; puffiness; dark circles under eyes; cellulite.*
The Liver	*If your liver is overloaded you may suffer from bloating, nausea, indigestion, and a furred tongue.*
The Lungs	*catarrh, runny nose or constant sneezing, clogged sinuses.*
The Kidneys	*dark-coloured, cloudy, scanty, or strong-smelling urine; pain when urinating.*
The Skin	*cellulite; congested, blotchy skin; blackheads, whiteheads, or pimples.*
The Intestines	*constipation, gas, and wind.*

Healthy food, healthy body

But what *is* good food? Every expert has a different theory as to what we should be eating. Should we be food combining or eating a raw "caveman" diet? Should we search out organic food or are we wasting our time and money? The first point to realize is that we are all different and our bodies need varying regimes. What suits my body might be anathema to yours. In China all food is served warm; in India you would eat raw, lightly cooked or highly spiced food according to your body-mind type.

Finding the right diet for you will be a case of trial and error. Most of us know instinctively which foods suit us and which methods of preparation our bodies like best.

However, there are certain guidelines on which virtually every expert and every system of holistic health agrees. These points form the bedrock of good nutrition. Follow them and your body will thank you.

GUIDELINES FOR HEALTHY EATING

The first thing to do is be positive. Buy and cook fresh food. If you can, choose organic vegetables, fruit, and meat. Non-organic produce is often treated to make it last longer and appear fresh. Always peel or skin non-organic vegetables and fruit to remove superficial additives. Fresh fish is a healthy option, too – although seafood can be contaminated by coastal pollution. Cooking fresh food need not take time and effort – grilling, poaching, stir-frying, and steaming are all speedy techniques. And choose locally produced food; it is less reliant on processing and additives to keep it looking fresh and appetizing.

Pick food in season wherever possible. Food grown and harvested at its natural pace will have the most nutrients and vitality. Food grown out of season is usually

HEALTHY FOODS
Fresh foods grown locally and organically contain the least toxins. Processed food, convenience meals, diet foods, confectionery, and soft drinks contain the most preservatives, colourings, and additives.

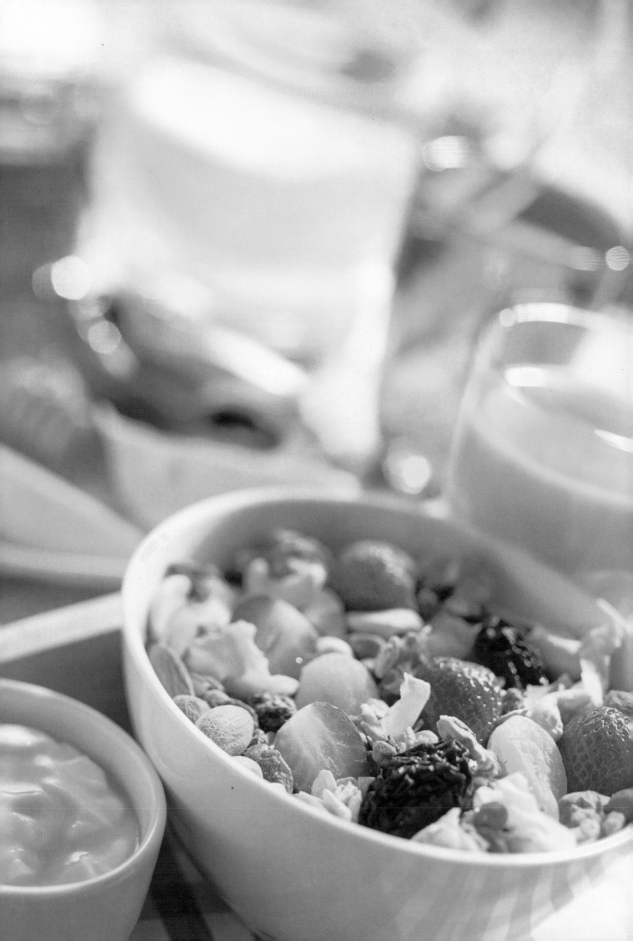

QUESTIONNAIRE ONE: FOOD AND DRINK

*In an ideal world you would score very low on this section – but we don't live in an ideal world!
Your body will probably be able to deal with a score under five – but don't expect to feel wonderful.
Between five and ten you are pushing your body and you can expect to have some chronic signs of
toxicity (allergies, tiredness, etc.). Upwards of ten you are putting your body under severe strain
and should seriously re-assess your nutrition.*

1 Do you drink coffee or tea regularly?   *yes* ☐ *no* ☐

2 Do you drink more than two glasses of wine, pints of beer or
spirit measures a day?   *yes* ☐ *no* ☐

3 Do you eat ready or convenience meals more than once a week?   *yes* ☐ *no* ☐

4 Do you eat a lot of processed (canned, frozen, dried, prepared) foods? *yes* ☐ *no* ☐

5 Do you eat much smoked produce; ie bacon, cheese, cooked meats?   *yes* ☐ *no* ☐

6 Do you add salt to your cooking or to your plate?   *yes* ☐ *no* ☐

7 Do you eat a lot of sugar, sweets, chocolates?   *yes* ☐ *no* ☐

8 Do you eat "diet" foods or use artificial sweeteners?   *yes* ☐ *no* ☐

9 Do you usually buy non-organic fruit, vegetables, meat?   *yes* ☐ *no* ☐

10 Do you eat a lot of processed meat products – burgers, sausages, pies? *yes* ☐ *no* ☐

11 Do you eat more than one fried meal a week?   *yes* ☐ *no* ☐

12 Do you drink a lot of sodas or fizzy drinks?   *yes* ☐ *no* ☐

13 Do you have take-outs or fast food meals more than once a week?   *yes* ☐ *no* ☐

14 Do you barbecue a lot of food (ie more than once a month?)   *yes* ☐ *no* ☐

15 Do you eat red meat more than once a week?   *yes* ☐ *no* ☐

Total ☐☐   ☐☐

forced with excess fertilizers and heavily treated with pesticides and fungicides. "Baby" or miniature vegetables will have been heavily treated, too.

Then cut down on your intake of red meat, full-fat dairy produce, and saturated fat. It is important to cut down on your salt intake, too. Don't add salt to your food, either when cooking or eating. Wean yourself off it by using herbs and spices, or adding celery which has a naturally salty taste.

Whenerever possible, avoid foods containing additives, colourings, and preservatives. This means all highly processed, convenience, and "junk" foods, including canned, dried, and packet foods plus ready-made meals and "fast foods". These foods, although tasty and tempting, contain a high proportion of chemical additives. If you suffer from asthma or other allergic conditions, be especially careful of additives. Children are also at much greater risk. So police your diet and cut out all processed foods. Simply by cutting out these foods, or by cutting them drastically from your diet, you will be taking huge steps towards better, safer health.

Avoid smoked meats and fish and steer clear of sausages and processed meats – they contain high levels of additives and potential carcinogens.

Be very wary of "diet" foods which often contain artificial sweeteners and other additives. If you are trying to lose weight, choose a simple low-fat, wholefood diet high in fresh vegetables, lean meat, nuts, and pulses. You will still lose weight – without compromising your health.

Cut out (or cut right down on) sweets. Most contain high levels of colourings, preservatives, and other additives. Unfortunately, children often have the worst reactions – brightly coloured sweets and soft drinks can often provoke hyperactivity and allergic reactions.

Genetic engineering

Foods that have been genetically engineered (GEs) are an almost totally unknown quantity. Experts say that genetic engineering of foods (altering their genetic structure to improve a particular quality) is an imprecise science with unpredictable outcomes.

PESTICIDES IN FOOD

Almost all non-organic food is grown with pesticides of some kind. Many are health-threatening; some are carcinogenic (they cause cancer); some may be mutagenic (mutating cells); others could be teratogenic (causing birth defects).

The worldwide death rate from pesticide poisonings alone tops 200,000 a year. A recent report found that pregnant women working with farm pesticides are almost three times as likely to lose their babies than other mothers-to-be. In 1993, a study showed that women with a high concentration of DDT (an infamous pesticide) residues in their bodies were four times more likely to develop breast cancer than other women. Yet we still keep spraying our crops.

It has been suggested that GEs may trigger more allergies such as asthma and skin problems. You might happily eat your bowl of strawberries and cream thinking you will be quite safe from your allergy to fish protein, not guessing for one moment that the strawberries have been manipulated with the gene of the Arctic sea flounder so they are more resistant to frost. Until we know more about genetically engineered food the obvious answer is for all of us to leave it out of our diets.

Irradiated food

Irradiation has been hailed as a wonderful new way of keeping food fresh for longer. Basically, the food is exposed to high doses of radiation which halt the growth of bacteria. Performed correctly it should not make food measurably radioactive but it does inevitably bring about chemical changes.

Irradiation breaks apart the molecules of food, which then form new molecules and new chemicals when they come back together again. The newly formed chemicals – called radiolytic products (RPs) and unique radiolytic products (URPs) do not exist in any foods except those irradiated. There has not been rigorous testing of these chemicals: the argument is that they are created in such tiny amounts that they couldn't possibly cause any harm. But who knows for sure?

CAFFEINE ADDICTION

Many of us rely on our morning coffee to wake us up. We drink tea or sodas throughout the day without a second thought. But all these contain caffeine, which is a powerful and addictive drug. Caffeine stresses the adrenal glands and puts our whole system in a state of unnatural alert. It is relatively easy to break the caffeine habit – but you may experience headaches, migraine, or irritability for a few days after giving up. If you can't give up, try cutting down – drink fewer cups; substitute herbal teas or coffee substitutes for a few cups; drink water or juice instead of soda. You will feel brighter, calmer, and clearer if you do.

WATER – VITAL FOR HEALTH

A staggering 70-75 per cent of our bodies is comprised of water. Drinking plenty of fresh, clean water is one of the most vital steps you can take for your health. Water helps the skin and kidneys to eliminate toxins; it also stimulates and flushes the liver. In addition, it softens the feces and helps waste pass more quickly through the gut, removing toxins. Ideally, we should be drinking around two litres (3.5 pints) of fresh water each day. Ayurvedic physicians recommend drinking water warm as this speeds the elimination of ama, or toxic waste. Simply boil fresh water for five minutes, put in a thermos flask, and drink at any time throughout the day.

Pure water

Water is essential to life but sadly our water supplies are often not as pure as they should be. Here are some ways to improve the water you use or cut down on the pollutants.

▪ If you can afford it, try a combined reverse osmosis and activated carbon unit. This can filter the water supply to the whole house.

▪ Much cheaper, and still quite effective, are activated carbon filters, in the form of plastic jugs you can keep in the refrigerator. However, they will not remove nitrates or dissolved metals such as iron, lead, or copper.

▪ If your water supply is unfiltered, try taking warm baths or cool showers rather than a piping hot shower. Many water-polluting chemicals can be vaporized in a hot shower – you might actually absorb up to 100 times more pollutants simply by breathing the air around a shower than drinking all the water that passes through it.

▪ Distilling water does remove many contaminants but those substances which have a boiling point very close to that of water, such as some of the trihalomethanes, cannot be removed. Do not store distilled water for long periods since bacteria breed very easily in it.

▪ Bottled water seems like a safe option. However, some brands of bottled water have been shown to have some 10,000 bacteria per millilitre. Choose bottled water in glass bottles rather than plastic containers.

Food sensitivities, allergies, and intolerances

Allergies and sensitivities are on the increase. One child in four now has a major allergy, which is a 400-500 per cent increase since the 1940s. Around 50 per cent of adults believe they are intolerant or allergic to certain foods. The prevalence of asthma alone is doubling every 20 years. There are many reasons touted for these extraordinary statistics but our toxic world certainly has a large part to play. Pollution has been linked to higher incidences of asthma and hay fever. And for many people, allergies are directly related to the diet they eat. Still more are highly sensitive to the additives in our food. Discover your food sensitivities and you could find many allergies improve or completely disappear.

There are basically two types of food allergies which are termed fixed and masked. Fixed food allergies produce an immediate, often severe, reaction and typically occur with peanuts, shellfish, and eggs. If you have a fixed food allergy, you will already know about it! Masked, or hidden, food allergies – commonly known as intolerances – are harder to detect as the reaction is milder and often cannot be associated with one particular food.

The month-long detox detailed in Chapter Four may well pinpoint your intolerances. The program cuts out the most common problem foods – wheat, dairy produce, sugar, coffee, tea, alcohol, and the additives in processed foods. If you introduce new foods one a day as you come off the program you may find some cause your old symptoms to return or give you headaches, palpitations, rashes, or anxiety attacks. If so, try cutting them out of your diet again and see if you improve.

If you still feel you have undetected intolerance problems after the one-month detox you should get the help of an experienced practitioner – so consult your physician, naturopath, or nutritional therapist.

ALLERGY CAUSING FOODS
Dairy produce, wheat, eggs, nuts, and shellfish are some of the problem foods that can cause food sensitivities, allergies, or intolerances.

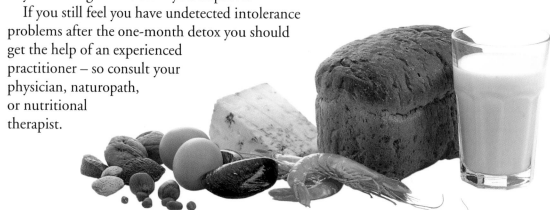

QUESTIONNAIRE TWO: FOOD SENSITIVITIES

Any of these symptoms could indicate a food allergy or sensitivity. If it is chronic and longstanding, it could be the result of the food you are eating. Once you discover what is causing the problem and eliminate it, results can seem almost miraculous. If a food is causing a serious allergy you may have to avoid it permanently. However, many people find they can reintroduce their problem foods, after desensitizing their bodies.

caution: *If you have a serious or chronic complaint you should always check with your physician.*

		yes	no
1	Do you suffer from: sneezing, runny nose, hay fever, or sinusitis?	☐	☐
2	Do you often wake up tired or feel weary or exhausted?	☐	☐
3	Do you have tender, sore, or bleeding gums; mouth ulcers; or a sore tongue?	☐	☐
4	Are there dark puffy circles under your eyes; do you bruise easily?	☐	☐
5	Do you suffer from frequent headaches, migraine, or dizziness?	☐	☐
6	Are you often irritable, tense, aggressive, or hyperactive?	☐	☐
7	Do you suffer from depression, confusion, or forgetfulness?	☐	☐
8	Are you very much over- or under-weight? Or does your weight constantly go up and down?	☐	☐
9	Do you suffer from eczema, urticaria, psoriasis, or acne?	☐	☐
10	Do you feel better for eating certain foods or drinks?	☐	☐
11	Do you crave particular foods or are you an obsessive eater?	☐	☐
12	Do you suffer from bloating, flatulence, indigestion?	☐	☐
13	Do you have either constipation or diarrhea?	☐	☐
14	Are you wheezy or breathless; do you have asthma?	☐	☐
15	Do you suffer from insomnia, waking in the night, or disturbed sleep?	☐	☐
16	Do your muscles ache or tingle?	☐	☐
17	Is your sex drive low?	☐	☐
18	Do you have painful or irregular periods; do you suffer from PMS?	☐	☐
19	Do your eyes water or itch a lot; are you very sensitive to bright lights?	☐	☐
20	Do you suffer palpitations, high or low blood pressure, or chest pains?	☐	☐

Total ☐☐ ☐☐

Clean environment, clear body

Now it's time to look at our home. You probably consider your home to be a refuge from the harsh and dangerous world. But, sadly, our homes too can be the cause of toxic overload. Recent reports indicate that we are exposed to up to 300 volatile organic (carbon-based) compounds within our homes. In America, the Environmental Protection Agency estimates that thousands of cancer deaths annually are brought about by indoor air pollutants – the hoard of chemicals which may be quietly seeping into our homes.

Indoor air pollutants range from dust, smoke, and airborne bacteria to the paints, cleaners, solvents, dyes, glues, and household sprays we use every day to clean and improve our homes. New curtains and carpets might be emitting formaldehyde gas, a highly toxic substance which causes serious health concerns. Home insulation may discharge man-made fibres, even asbestos, into the air we breathe. Pressed-wood and fibreboard furniture and fittings can emit harmful chemicals while electromagnetic radiation from household appliances like the TV, refrigerator, and even an electric blanket can also adversely affect our health.

Take a tour around your home and you will find toxic materials in the most surprising places. Products that seemed like a dream – carpets that wouldn't stain, furniture made from inexpensive pressed woods, wallpaper that wouldn't mould – are now filling our homes with a host of hazards.

NEW HOME HAZARDS

The newer your home and its furnishings, the more likely it is that your pollution levels will be higher:
- Roofing timbers may have been treated with toxic fluids or insulated with unhealthy materials.
- Cavity walls could have been injected with an insulating foam which emits formaldehyde.
- Paint releases solvents like toluene, xylene, and benzene (all potentially toxic) and could contain mercury (which may cause brain damage) as a fungicide.
- Wall-to-wall synthetic carpeting (plus its backing and padding) can emit toxins such as benzene, formaldehyde, toluene, zylene, and styrene.

SMOKING

Nicotine is a powerful drug which creates a huge dependency, so it's not surprising people find it desperately hard to give up smoking. But, if you can stop, you will be giving your body the greatest gift imaginable.

But how can you do it? First of all, you have to decide that you really do want to give up. Enlist the support of your family and friends. Seek professional help, too.

Several forms of holistic health can bring good results. Hypnotherapy, in which you work on your reasons for dependence, can be highly effective. Acupuncture can stop or ease the craving for nicotine and homeopathy can also help people kick the habit.

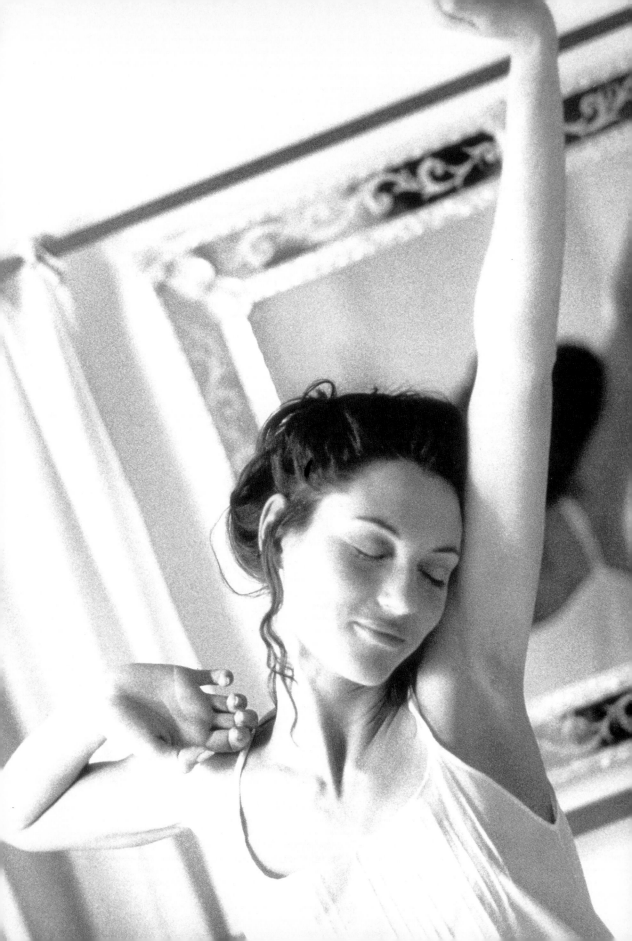

QUESTIONNAIRE THREE: YOUR HOME ENVIRONMENT

Questions 1-5 deal with the environment surrounding your home. If you answer yes to one or more questions here you may have high levels of external pollution. Keep your body as healthy as possible by regularly detoxing. If you have answered yes to question 5 get your home checked for radon (see p. 26). Questions 6-12 deal with the fabric, decoration, and furnishings of your home. Several yes answers here and you need to take active steps to reduce your internal toxic overload. Yes answers to questions 13-16 indicate that the products you're using may be contributing to your toxic home.

1   Do you live within a mile of a major road or highway?   *yes* ☐   *no* ☐

2   Do high voltage overhead power cables run within half a mile of your home?   *yes* ☐   *no* ☐

3   Do you live in an area where fields are routinely sprayed?   *yes* ☐   *no* ☐

4   Are you living under or near a flight path?   *yes* ☐   *no* ☐

5   Do you live in an area with a lot of granite, shale, or sedimentary rock?   *yes* ☐   *no* ☐

6   Does your home have cavity wall insulation?   *yes* ☐   *no* ☐

7   Is your plumbing more than 20 years old?   *yes* ☐   *no* ☐

8   Has your home been treated for woodworm or rot in the last five years, or have you put in new timber?   *yes* ☐   *no* ☐

9   Does your home contain a lot of old paintwork (ie 20 years or more) – or have you recently painted your home?   *yes* ☐   *no* ☐

10   Have you recently had new synthetic carpets or vinyl flooring laid?   *yes* ☐   *no* ☐

11   Do you have curtains or furniture covered in synthetic fabrics, particularly those with "stain resistant" finishes?   *yes* ☐   *no* ☐

12   Do you have much chipboard, fibreboard, plywood, or MDF in your home?   *yes* ☐   *no* ☐

13   Do you have your clothes dry-cleaned regularly?   *yes* ☐   *no* ☐

14   Do you commonly use pesticides in your home and garden?   *yes* ☐   *no* ☐

15   Do you use large amounts of bleach, detergent, household cleaners, disinfectant?   *yes* ☐   *no* ☐

16   Do you use synthetic (and particularly aerosol) air fresheners?   *yes* ☐   *no* ☐

Total ☐☐   ☐☐

■ Furniture coverings and curtains made from synthetic fibres can emit noxious chemicals such as vinyl chloride, styrene, and formaldehyde.

■ Paintwork in older homes may have high levels of lead, which can be extremely toxic, or asbestos, which is well-known for its serious health risks. The asbestos may be found as insulation for hot water and steam pipes, heat ducts, and furnaces. It is also found in wall insulation, roofing, and siding. In the 1960s and 1970s, it was even used in some curtain fabrics.

UNSEEN DANGERS IN OUR HOMES

The fuels we use for cooking and heating (gas, paraffin, kerosene, oil, coal, and wood) can all release harmful by-products into the air of our homes. These may build up to dangerous levels indoors, especially if you live in a so-called "tight" house – a home with super-insulated walls and ceilings. Such homes may be warm, cosy, and cheap to run but they exchange indoor air as little as twice daily while an adequate level is considered to be three times as high. All the hazardous fumes and gases are left to circulate, and we breathe them in.

Gas cookers and boilers produce large amounts of carbon monoxide, carbon dioxide, nitric oxide, and nitrogen dioxide, as well as smaller amounts of formaldehyde, sulphur dioxide, and other by-products.

Portable paraffin (kerosene) and gas heaters are unvented and so are particularly hazardous. Even the archetypal home fire, quietly burning coal or logs, can pump pollutants, particularly carbon monoxide, into the home. Most goes up the chimney but, if your flue is unswept, cracked, or inefficient, toxic gases can re-enter your living room. Believe it or not but wood smoke is also a suspected carcinogen.

TOXIC HOUSEWORK

So far we've only talked about the dangers in the very fabric and furnishings of the home. But there is another troop of toxins we willingly import into the home in our shopping bags: the tools of housework. Modern polishes, detergents, fabric and carpet cleaners, air fresheners and

ELECTROMAGNETISM

All electrical appliances give off electromagnetic radiation. Although the levels from household equipment (TVs, computers, microwaves, hairdryers, etc.) are low, research indicates that electromagnetic fields (EMFs) may cause insomnia, high blood pressure, anxiety, and general ill-health. They can also trigger allergic reactions, headaches, and nausea.

Minimize the use of electrical appliances, keeping them switched off when not in use. In particular, keep them out of your bedroom: never fall asleep watching TV or with your computer left running.

oven cleaners make keeping the home clean and fresh a much simpler task than in the past. But while they may take the elbow-grease out of cleaning, they put in a host of hazards that may harm you and harm the environment. Many contain potentially harmful VOCs (volatile organic compounds). These chemicals release vapours into the air that may be toxic and are often certainly irritant. Aerosols can dispense harmful irritants in a fine mist which is easily absorbed either by breathing it into the lungs or through the skin – or both.

The key here is to simplify your cleaning. It isn't necessary to use so many high-tech chemical products: there are simple natural alternatives to chemical housekeeping. Also, health stores and some supermarkets now stock "green" products which are friendly to the environment as well as protecting our health.

HOME AND GARDEN PESTICIDES

Perhaps the most lethal substances present in many of our homes are chemicals that are specifically designed to kill pests. "Pests" include a huge number of insects and some mammals: flies, wasps and bees, aphids, mice, rats, slugs, and even birds. It seems that for every pest or combination of pests we might encounter, there is a pesticide, insecticide, dusting powder, or spray of some kind that will eliminate the problem.

There are several hundred household and garden pest control products on the market, most of which contain powerful chemical ingredients which upset the natural order of wildlife. Many will pose a threat to your health. Pest control products may, for instance, cause irritation or allergic reaction, including headache, cold symptoms, rashes, sore eyes, and throat. They can be very poisonous – in fact, some are fatal to us and/or our pets. Some may cause cancer, genetic mutation, or birth defects in humans and animals.

HELPFUL PLANTS

*One simple, effective, and very pleasant way to deal with environmental toxins is to fill your home and office with house plants. Remarkable research by NASA found that certain species can actually remove pollutants such as formaldehyde, benzene, and trichloroethylene from the air. Golden pothos (*Scindapsus aureus*), nephthytis (*Syngonium podophyllum*) and the spider plant (*Chlorophytum elatum vittatum*) can all remove substantial amounts of chemical contamination. Other research suggests philodendrons may be even more effective.*

QUESTIONNAIRE FOUR: YOUR WORKPLACE ENVIRONMENT

High scores in questions 1-4 means your workplace is a probably a "sick" building or that you are particularly sensitive to the environment. Questions 6-10 concern additional problems in the workplace – unfortunately they are hard to avoid – but you can take measures to protect yourself. Questions 11-13 consider the impact of commuting and travelling – if you score highly here you will have an additional toxic burden. The last two questions concern mental toxicity – a factor often forgotten in the workplace. If work is unduly stressful, focus on techniques for coping with tension and anxiety.

1 Do you suffer from the symptoms of ill-health, which go away when you leave the workplace and return when you return? *yes* ☐ *no* ☐

2 Do the symptoms get worse when the heat or air conditioning is turned on? *yes* ☐ *no* ☐

3 Did you start feeling bad when you moved into a new office or when your workplace was redecorated or remodelled? Or when lagging, cavity foam, etc. was installed in the workplace? *yes* ☐ *no* ☐

4 Do the symptoms become more severe when the workplace is tightly sealed in cold weather? *yes* ☐ *no* ☐

5 Do you have to use toxic chemicals or their by-products as part of your work? *yes* ☐ *no* ☐

6 Do you use a lot of commercial detergents, cleaners, paint, etc.? *yes* ☐ *no* ☐

7 Do you work on a computer for more than an hour a day? *yes* ☐ *no* ☐

8 Are there many electrical or electronic machines operating near you – ie photocopiers, computers, processors? *yes* ☐ *no* ☐

9 Do people smoke in your workplace? *yes* ☐ *no* ☐

10 Do you work under fluorescent lights? Do you have no natural lighting in your workplace? *yes* ☐ *no* ☐

11 Does your work involve driving long distance – ie more than 60 miles a day? *yes* ☐ *no* ☐

12 Do you take a lot of flights, and particularly long distance flights – ie more than two a year? *yes* ☐ *no* ☐

13 Do you have to travel through a city centre on your way to work? *yes* ☐ *no* ☐

14 Is your work very stressful? Do you often find yourself feeling anxious or panicked? *yes* ☐ *no* ☐

15 Do you dread going to work in the morning? *yes* ☐ *no* ☐

Total ☐☐ ☐☐

HOW TO SAFEGUARD YOUR HOUSE

Don't be discouraged if you have scored highly in this
section. Most modern homes have a high degree of
toxicity. However, once we know where the dangers lie we
can take simple steps to minimize – or eliminate – them.
- Keep your house well-aired. Open all the windows for
at least fifteen minutes each morning and evening. Use
exhaust fans in kitchens and bathrooms.
- Wherever you can, choose non-toxic building materials
for repairs and new work. Ensure all decorating materials
and new furnishings you buy have not been treated with
dangerous chemicals.
- Regularly service all your heaters and boilers to reduce
carbon monoxide leakage. For those who like to have an
open fire, make sure you sweep the flue regularly and keep
the room well-aired while in use.
- Organize professionals to remove old lead paint and
asbestos. Don't attempt to do this yourself.
- Unwrap dry-cleaned clothes and leave them in the open
air for a few hours before hanging in your wardrobe.
- Buy ionizers, air purifiers, or combined ionizer/purifiers
– particularly if you have answered yes to any of questions
6-12 in the questionnaire on page 22.
- Instal a water purification system for your domestic
water supply.
- Replace fluorescent lighting: typical health complaints
include nausea, eyestrain, headaches, depression, and even
panic attacks. Use daylight bulbs – especially if you suffer
from SAD (seasonal affective disorder).

RADON

Radon is a natural radioactive gas which seeps up into
houses through gaps in floors and walls; it damages lung
tissue and causes 2,500 deaths each year in the UK alone
from lung cancer.

   Local authorities and environmental health
organizations can help determine if you have a radon
problem and may give financial assistance in curing it.
Radon can be prevented from seeping into your home
by building a suspended concrete floor or under-floor
fans beneath the building can suck the gas away.

GEOPATHIC STRESS

Abnormal energy fields generated by deep underground streams, large mineral deposits, or faults in the substrata of the earth can produce geopathic stress (GS). Odd as it may seem, GS can be a contributing factor in everything from migraines to cancer, from nightmares to divorce.

In Germany it has been researched since the 1920s and is taken very seriously. Experiments have shown that bacteria grow abnormally over underground currents of water while mice inoculated with disease will fall ill far more rapidly when kept over a subterranean vein of water. Now builders in Germany and Austria test sites for GS before building and many will routinely give guarantees that new buildings do not have lines of "bad" energy passing through them.

However, even if your house does suffer GS, your health need not necessarily be affected. GS comes up through the earth in thin bands or small spirals so will only affect you if you are sleeping directly on top of it or sitting in it all day.

DETECTING GEOPATHIC STRESS

If you suspect geopathic stress might be affecting your home try detecting it yourself:
- *Do you or anyone in your home constantly feel tired and below par? Is everything an effort? Are you easily depressed and irritable? Do you constantly suffer from colds while illnesses, aches, and pains will not respond to any treatment? Do children become unaccountably disruptive and badly behaved?*
- *Because GS comes up through the earth in thin bands it can easily affect just one person in the house – a band can pass through one side of a bed or one armchair. Only one member of the family could be affected.*
- *If you suspect you suffer from GS, try putting cork tiles under your bed or favourite chair for a few weeks to see whether you start to feel better. The tiles seem to neutralize the rays for a limited period. If you do start to feel better, try moving your bed or chair.*
- *Watch where your pets sleep. Cats adore GS and will often sleep on a bad spot while dogs will avoid it at all costs. If the cat always makes straight for your favourite armchair, try moving it to the dog's favourite spot.*
- *Babies are apparently very sensitive to GS. If your baby constantly rolls over to one corner of the cot he or she may be attempting to escape GS. Move the cot to another part of the room and see whether the baby stays where it is put.*
- *If you feel you are affected by GS try the following: switch on a hairdryer and run it all over you with the side of the dryer touching your body. It sounds crazy but try it once a week – it does appear to help.*

Chapter Two

Body detox exercises

Choose and develop your own physical detox program from a whole host of exercises, workouts, and activities – from aerobics, yoga, chi kung, and rebounding to cycling, tai chi, Pilates, and swimming.

Nature intended us to be active. We were not designed to sit at desks all day; to be cramped into cars; to peer at computer screens. In this chapter we're going to look at simple and straightforward ways to help you detox through movement. I'm not going to suggest you start running marathons – good exercise starts with something as non-threatening as good breathing! After that, we will look at ways you can start to introduce movement into your everyday life. Exercise for detoxing is not about sporting prowess or pumping increasing amounts of iron: even its most gentle forms can be deceptively effective.

But how does exercise help the detox process? Aerobic exercise (which increases your heart rate above normal and keeps it there for a continuous amount of time) helps improve your circulation, strengthens the heart and lungs, and enables them to work more efficiently. It also increases oxygenation so you have a better exchange of gases at a cellular level. By working your muscles, you also help the lymphatic system pump more effectively. There are psychological benefits, too. Tough aerobic exercise is one way of dispersing the excess stress hormones so our bodies and minds can return to a relaxed state.

Non-aerobic exercises, such as yoga, tai chi, and chi kung, are equally effective in helping us detox. They stretch and tone not only the muscles but also the major organs and body systems. This gentle exercise stimulates the lymph just as effectively as "hard" aerobics. These more meditative forms of exercise work on the nervous system, refreshing the body and calming the mind.

Of the enormous variety of sports, exercises, and techniques available to help you detox, there will be one for you, whatever your age, inclination, or state of fitness!

MOTIVATION

■ *How do you like to exercise? In private? Use equipment at home, follow techniques on video, or try running, walking, cycling, etc. On your own but surrounded by others? Join a gym or class. With a partner? Find someone to exercise with. As part of a team? Look out for team sports or clubs. With an instructor? Join a gym or invest in a personal trainer.*

■ *Schedule your workout times as firm dates in your diary and keep to them. Working out with others provides incentive – it's often harder to let them down than yourself!*

■ *Your chosen exercise needs to be easily accessible so you can make it part of your daily life.*

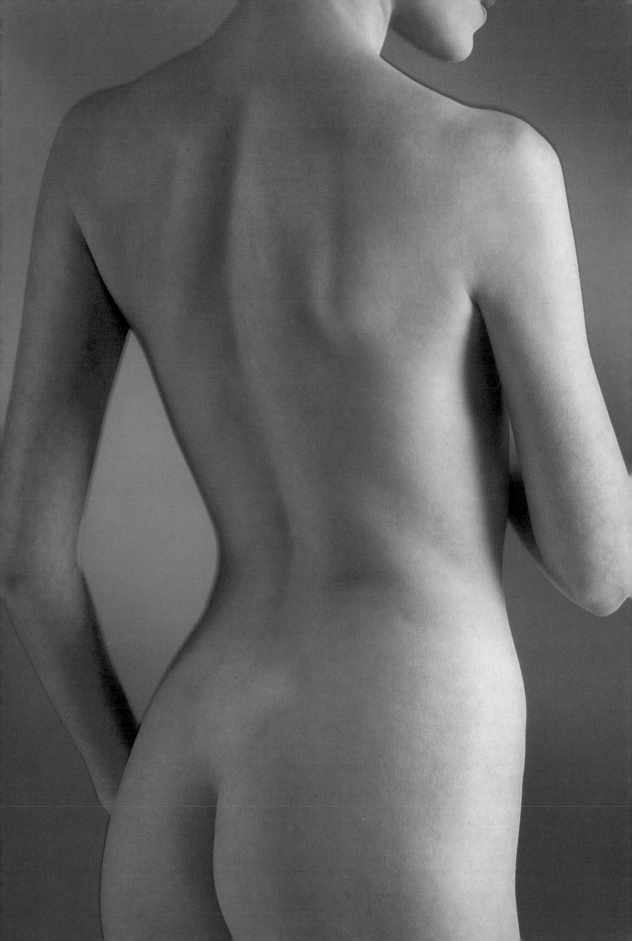

Breathing your body clean

Breathing is the way we pull in oxygen and circulate it around the body to "feed" each and every cell; it is also the way we send out carbon dioxide and waste products, "cleaning out" each and every cell. The more oxygen you can get around your body, the better; the more effectively you can clear waste from your body, the better. Breathing fully can do everything from improving your moods, increasing your resistance to colds and illness, fostering better sleep, and even helping you resist aging. It feeds the brain, calms the nerves, and has a measurable effect on a number of medical conditions – lowering heart rate and metabolic rate, normalizing blood pressure, and decreasing the risks of cardiovascular disease.

Basically, almost all of us breathe too shallowly, only using a tiny portion of our lungs. When we inhale we only take in around a glassful of air when we could, in fact, take in at least three times that amount.

The lungs are made up of around 700 million air sacs of which the greater proportion lie in the lower lungs. When we breathe shallowly, we don't ever quite expel all the waste gases and detritus in the lower lungs. We also run the risk of losing vital elasticity in the lower part of our lungs.

Fortunately, there are very simple exercises which can help bring our breathing back to its optimum fullness and freedom. The yogic tradition of India developed a whole science of breathing. They called it pranayama, the science of breath control and expansion.

In China, the effects of the breathing which forms an integral part of chi kung have been rigorously tested. Experiments have shown that chi kung exercises can increase lung capacity from an average of 428.5 cubic centimetres to 561.8 (26.14 to 34.27 cubic inches).

On a symbolic level, breathing is all about detoxing – taking in the new and eliminating the old. The Buddhist tradition regards every new breath as giving new life and every exhalation as a little death. Taking in deep joyful breaths is seen as a way of affirming life and vitality. Breathing minimally and shallowly is, in a way, turning your back on life or accepting it only grudgingly. There is a yoga proverb which says: "Life is in the breath. Therefore he who only half breathes, half lives."

CAUTION

The breathing exercises of chi kung and pranayama can be very powerful processes. Anyone with a chest problem should take the exercises very slowly and carefully, preferably under the guidance of a trained teacher. Anyone with a heart condition, blood pressure problem, or glaucoma should not hold the breath – again consult a trained teacher. If in any doubt, consult your physician or a trained practitioner.

THE COMPLETE BREATH

This is the basic breathing technique of pranayama. It is an
excellent training tool as it encourages you to breathe fully,
bringing oxygen deep into the cells and pulling out toxins.

1 *Lie down on the floor and make yourself comfortable.
Bring your feet close in to your buttocks and allow the feet
to fall apart. Bring the soles together, resting your hands
gently on your abdomen. (If this feels uncomfortable put
cushions under your knees.) This posture stretches the
lower abdomen, which enhances the breathing process.*

2 *Breathe in slowly and smoothly
through your nostrils, conscious of
the breath as it moves through your
chest. Feel your abdomen expand
and your fingers part.*

3 *Exhale slowly and steadily
through your nostrils, noticing
your abdomen flatten and your
fingers are once again touching.
After a pause, repeat this cycle
and breathe at your own pace
for five minutes or as long as
you feel comfortable.*

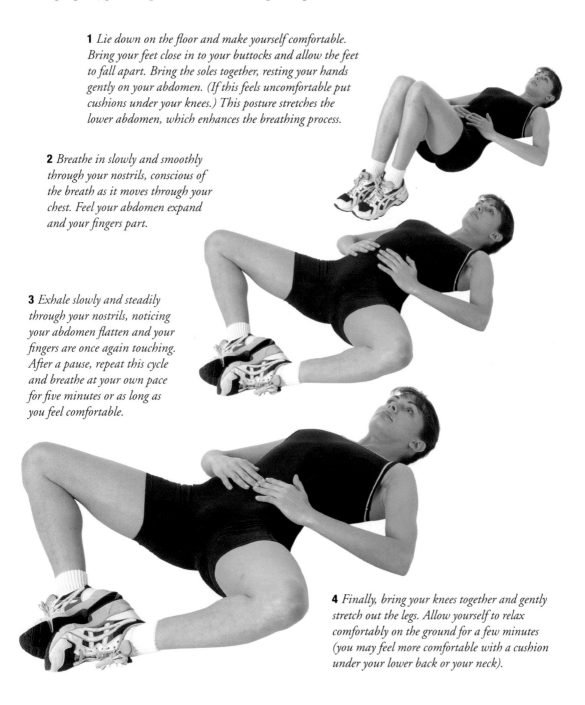

4 *Finally, bring your knees together and gently
stretch out the legs. Allow yourself to relax
comfortably on the ground for a few minutes
(you may feel more comfortable with a cushion
under your lower back or your neck).*

NOSTRIL BREATHING

This classic pranayama technique feels rather strange to begin with but, once you become used to it, is very soothing. It is particularly useful if you are feeling stressed or anxious – or if you cannot sleep at night.

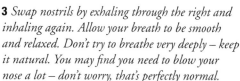

1 Sit comfortably in a chair, with both feet on the floor. Don't slouch. Then gently allow your eyes to close, your body to relax, and your mind to still.

Place your dominant hand around your nose. If you are right-handed, place your right thumb against your right nostril and let the fingers lie gently towards your left nostril. The aim is to close off one nostril at a time, comfortably and easily, without constantly moving your hand.

2 Close the right nostril gently and slowly exhale through your left nostril. Note that you are starting the breath on an exhale. Then inhale through the same nostril.

3 Swap nostrils by exhaling through the right and inhaling again. Allow your breath to be smooth and relaxed. Don't try to breathe very deeply – keep it natural. You may find you need to blow your nose a lot – don't worry, that's perfectly normal.

4 Alternate between the two nostrils for around five minutes. If you feel uncomfortable at any time, breathe through your mouth for a while until you can go back to the nose. When you've finished, simply sit and relax with your eyes closed for a few moments.

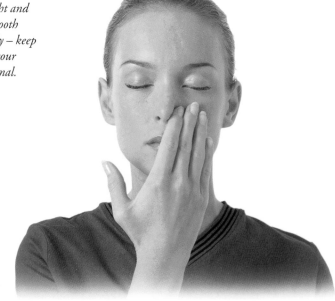

DETOX BREATH

This is a superb breathing exercise which will help improve elimination of toxins. It strengthens the lungs, massages and tones the abdominal muscles, and refreshes the nervous system. However, it should not be used if you have a heart condition, high blood pressure, epilepsy, hernia, or any ear, nose, or eye problems. **See note**, *right*, **if you are pregnant or menstruating.**

note: *If you are pregnant or menstruating try a much slower form of the detox breath. Instead of the "sneezing" exhale, pout your lips and allow your breath to come out through in a steady stream, as if you were blowing out candles on a cake. This is good for calming down in a difficult situation.*

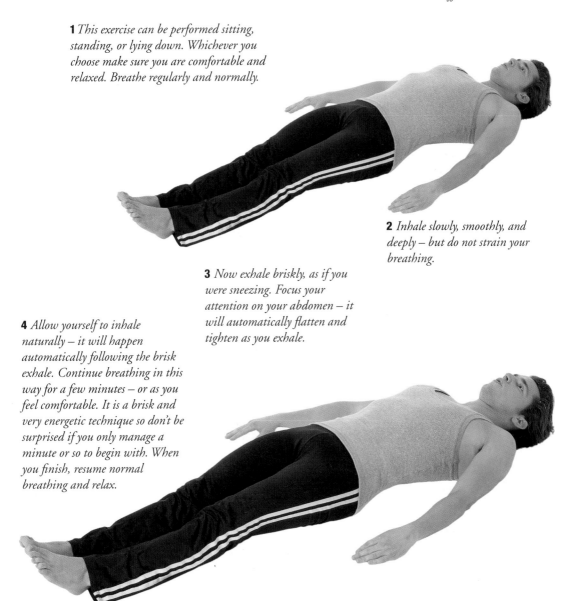

1 *This exercise can be performed sitting, standing, or lying down. Whichever you choose make sure you are comfortable and relaxed. Breathe regularly and normally.*

2 *Inhale slowly, smoothly, and deeply – but do not strain your breathing.*

3 *Now exhale briskly, as if you were sneezing. Focus your attention on your abdomen – it will automatically flatten and tighten as you exhale.*

4 *Allow yourself to inhale naturally – it will happen automatically following the brisk exhale. Continue breathing in this way for a few minutes – or as you feel comfortable. It is a brisk and very energetic technique so don't be surprised if you only manage a minute or so to begin with. When you finish, resume normal breathing and relax.*

Stretching

A stretched body is a supple, flexible, healthy body. Stretching is simplicity itself yet it offers a host of benefits to both body and mind. If you carry out a careful stretch routine before and after exercise or sports, you are far less likely to suffer from injury. It's also essential if you spend your days stuck at a desk or behind the wheel of a car: stretching can release stress and unwind tense muscles.

Best of all for our detox purposes, stretching helps the body to throw out toxins by increasing oxygenation and stimulating lymphatic drainage. As a huge bonus (and a definite incentive!), a well-stretched body looks great: lean and elegant. Your posture should improve and you will be far less likely to suffer neck, shoulder, and back pain, or headaches and bad digestion. Apart from all this, stretching feels simply wonderful and is an excellent way to get back in touch with your body.

Virtually anyone can follow a simple stretch routine – you don't need to be super-fit or agile. However, if you suffer from a bad back you should seek professional advice before stretching.

This simple stretch routine covers all the major muscle groups of the body. Try to make it a daily habit. You should always stretch before and after energetic exercise so incorporate this into your workouts. It is also a wonderful way to wind down after a long day at work or whenever you find yourself feeling tired and stressed.

SIMPLE STRETCH ROUTINE

The sequence of stretches on the following pages make up a simple routine for you to incorporate into your everyday schedule. You can wear shoes but it is much better to perform the stretches barefoot. Wear loose comfortable clothes if you can.

Take the stretches slowly and carefully: don't over-stretch. The idea is to feel the stretch but not to give yourself any discomfort or pain. Don't "bounce" the stretch to make it more intense: once in the pose, hold it without movement. And come out of the stretch slowly not abruptly. If you cannot achieve the full stretch, go as far as you can. You will find that, with practice, you can swiftly increase your flexibility.

‣ CALF STRETCH

*Stand a little distance away from a wall, cross
your arms and lean them against the wall. Now
lean your forehead against your hands. Bend your
left knee and extend your right leg out behind you.
Keep both feet parallel, pointing straight ahead.
Slowly move your hips forwards, keeping your
feet flat, until you feel a slight stretch in the calf
muscles of the extended leg. Hold gently for a
slow count of ten. Now change legs and repeat.*

‣ QUADRICEPS AND KNEE STRETCH

*Keeping one hand on the wall for support,
reach behind your back with your left
hand and grasp your right foot by the toes.
Keep your supporting knee softly bent; tuck
your pelvis forwards and stand up straight.
Hold gently for a count of 20 and release.
Now do the same with the opposite hand
and foot.*

‹ GROIN STRETCH

*Sit on the floor with the soles of your feet
together. Put your hands on your feet and
pull your heels in towards your body. This is
a strong stretch so don't worry if you can't get
very far at first. Now gently pull your body
forwards, towards your feet, keeping your back
erect until you feel a stretch. Hold for a count
of 20. As you hold the stretch, concentrate on
relaxing your arms, shoulders, and feet.*

◄ HAMSTRINGS STRETCH

Still sitting, straighten your right leg out in front of you. Keep your left leg bent, bringing the sole to face the inside of the right leg (as far as you can). Keep the right leg slightly bent. With your hands relaxed on the floor, bend forwards slightly from the hips until you feel an easy stretch. Touch the top of the thigh of your right leg and check it is feeling soft and relaxed. Keep your foot upright, not turned out. Hold for a count of 30. Release and repeat with your left leg.

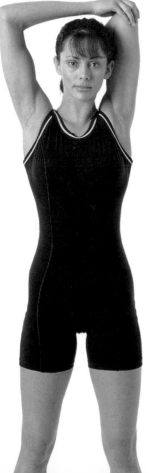

▸ UPPER HAMSTRINGS AND HIP STRETCH

With your left leg extended in front of you, bend your right leg and bring it up towards your abdomen, cradling it in your arms like a baby. Gently pull the leg towards you until you feel an easy stretch. Hold for a count of 20, release, and then repeat with the other leg.

◄ ARM STRETCH

Bring yourself gently to your feet. Raise your left arm up above your head. Grasp it at the elbow with your right hand. Now let your left hand drop down behind your shoulder blade (or as far as you can go). Gently pull the left arm back and in towards the head. Keep your arm, neck, and shoulders relaxed. Hold for a count of 20 then release and repeat on the other side.

▸ ARCH STRETCH

Sit on your toes (kneeling but so you are resting your buttocks on your heels with your toes on the floor). Keep your hands on the floor in front of you for balance. Gently stretch the arches of the feet. Hold for a count of 10.

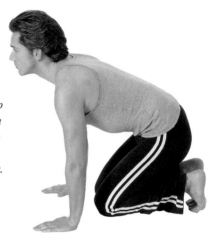

1 ▾ ALL-OVER STRETCH

Stand upright with your feet shoulder width apart, feet facing forwards. Extend your arms in front of you at chest height with palms touching.

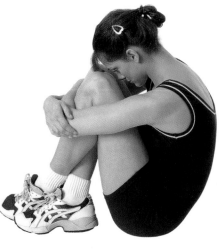

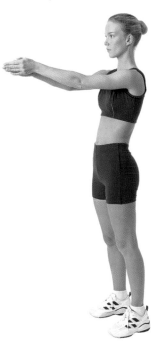

▴ BACK STRETCH

Sit down and bring your knees up to your chest (with your ankles crossed). Clasp your knees with both arms. Drop your head down to your knees and roll backwards on your spine. Roll forwards and backwards several times.

2 ▸ *Now bring your arms slowly back and down; then on behind your back. Clasp your hands behind your back with your arms extended straight down (hands in line with your buttocks). Now inhale deeply, pulling your shoulders back.*

3 ▸ *Exhale and bend forwards, raising your arms (still clasped at the hands) over your head.*

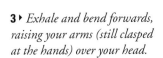

4 ▸ *Return very slowly to an upright position with your arms held loosely behind your back with hands clasped. Now slowly twist to the right and then to the left. Repeat the whole stretch three times.*

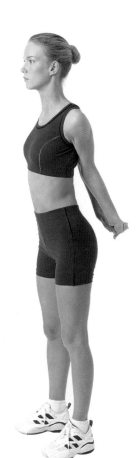

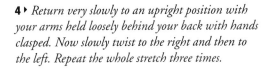

Yoga – the master exercise

Yoga puts pressure on all the different organs and muscles of the body very systematically. It tones the whole inner body as well as the outer body: the liver, the lungs, the kidneys, the spleen, the intestines, the heart. So it's not surprising that it is a detox exercise par excellence.

Yoga teachers claim that the precise asanas (postures) of yoga work far into the body – causing blood to circulate deeply rather than just around the periphery of the body, nourishing every organ and softening the muscle and ligament tissue. The deep stretching is said to bring both bones and muscles gently back into their optimum alignment while lubricating the joints.

Yoga can increase the oxygenation of your blood, improve circulation, and maximize the discharge of toxins – without having to sustain a high heart-rate as in typical aerobic exercise.

Not only does the body detox while you perform yoga; your mind does, too. The breathing directly affects the nervous system, eliciting the "relaxation response" in which the parasympathetic nervous system takes over from the sympathetic nervous system so that you feel calm, cool, and in control.

WHICH KIND OF YOGA SHOULD YOU CHOOSE?

There are almost as many different kinds of yoga as there are days in the year. The following are the ones you are most likely to come across.

- *Iyengar yoga: a very focused precise form of yoga which puts great emphasis on correct postures.*

- *Ashtanga yoga (also called Ashtanga Vinyassa yoga): the so-called "power" yoga puts very strong emphasis on sequences of postures, often carried out at much greater speed than the other forms of yoga. This is as close to aerobics as yoga gets.*

- *Sivananda yoga: a gentle, laid-back form of yoga.*

- *Vini yoga: puts emphasis on individual tuition. Safe and gentle.*

- *Dru yoga: expect to work with other people, including the whole group. A very gentle, holistic approach which includes pranayama (breath-work), deep relaxation, and meditation.*

- *Mana yoga: uses asanas (postures) alongside meditation, energy balancing, and creative visualization.*

The box on the opposite page gives you an idea of the range of yoga available. However, most classes will contain much the same elements: putting the body into specific postures and holding them for some time (except for Ashtanga yoga); breathing exercises (usually incorporated into the postures but some classes will also teach the art of breathing – pranayama – separately); and relaxation (sometimes with visualization). Some classes will also teach meditation and chanting. If you are unsure what to expect from a class, talk to the tutor before you join or ask to sit in and watch a class in progress.

THE SUN SALUTE

The Sun Salute, or Salutation to the Sun, is a well-known yoga routine (see pp. 40-41). It is deservedly becoming popular as it is perhaps the most effective series of exercises you can do for your body. It systematically stretches virtually every muscle in your body and massages the internal organs as well.

In ancient India the Salutation to the Sun was part of daily spiritual practice and was performed in the very early morning facing the sun, the deity for health and long life.

The benefits of regular practice with just this one exercise are legion. You will become far more flexible, particularly in your spine. You will increase your breathing capacity and help the elimination of toxins. It can even help reduce a fat tummy. There are 12 spinal positions and each stretches different ligaments and moves the spine in different ways.

At first, this series of exercises will seem jerky and uncoordinated – but persevere! As you begin to learn them off by heart you will find you can move fluidly and smoothly from one to another. Start off with just one whole set and gradually build up to the optimum 12. You may find it helpful to record the instructions on a tape recorder until you become familiar with them.

CAUTIONS

Just like any form of exercise yoga can harm as well as heal – if you practice it incorrectly.
- *Beginners should always go to a teacher, not a book or video.*
- *Find a well-qualified teacher – see Resources on page 122.*
- *Don't push yourself too far too fast. Yoga is not competitive – everyone works at their own pace. You will soon find you can stretch further or work harder.*
- *If you have a health problem (particularly a heart condition, back problem, or if you have recently had an operation), look for a yoga therapist (who has had a strict medical training) rather than a yoga teacher.*
- *Tell your teacher about any health or fitness problems you have. Find out which postures to avoid and which may help.*
- *If pregnant you will need to avoid certain postures. See a yoga therapist or find a class designed for pregnant women.*

2 Inhale slowly and deeply while you bring your arms straight up over your head, placing your palms together as you finish inhaling. Gently look back towards your thumbs. Lift the knees by tightening your thighs. Reach up as far as possible, lengthening your body. If you feel you can, take the posture back slightly further into a bend.

1 Stand upright, bring your feet together so the big toes are touching, and let your arms hang beside you. Relax your shoulders and tuck your chin in slightly – look straight ahead. Bring your hands together in front of your chest with palms together as if you were praying. Exhale deeply.

3 Exhale as you bend forwards so that your hands are in line with your feet. Your head should touch your knees. To begin with you may have to bend your knees in order to reach. You should eventually be able to straighten your knees into the full posture.

4 Inhale deeply and move your left leg away from your body in a big backwards sweep so you end up in a kind of extended lunge position. Keep your hands and right foot firmly on the ground. Bend your head upwards, stretching out your back.

5 Exhaling deeply bring yourself into an arched position. Keep your arms shoulder-width apart, and place your hands on the ground, palms facing directly in front. Your back, head, and arms should be in a straight line. Keep your feet and heels flat on the floor.

6 Exhale and lower your body onto the floor. Only eight parts of your body should touch the ground: feet, knees, hands, chest, and forehead. Keep your abdomen raised and, if you can, keep your nose off the floor so only your forehead makes contact. Don't worry if it's impossible – just keep the idea in mind.

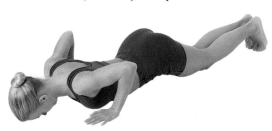

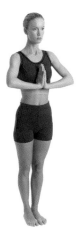

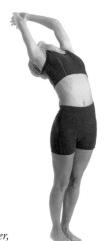

11 ◂ *Raise your arms over your head and bend backwards as you inhale (as for posture two).*

10 ◂ *Exhale and return to posture three.*

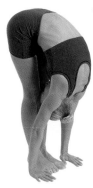

12 ▴ *Return to a comfortable standing position, feet together, arms by your sides. Look straight ahead and exhale. To close, bring your hands back together in a position of prayer.*

9 ▸ *Inhale and return to posture four, this time with the opposite leg forwards. So your left foot is in line with your hands while your right leg is stretched back.*

7 ▾ *Inhale and bend up into the position known as the cobra. Hands on the floor in front of you, arms straight, and bend backwards as far as feels comfortable. Look upwards.*

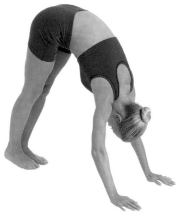

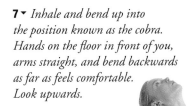

8 ▴ *Exhale and lift your back into the position five (known as the dog). Remember to keep your feet and heels (if you can) flat on the floor.*

Chi kung

Chi kung (also known as qi gong) is a holistic system that combines breathing techniques with precise movements and mental concentration: its aim is total health and wellbeing. Chi kung means "internal energy exercise" and is a simple and effective addition to your detoxing armoury. Practise chi kung daily – preferably in loose comfortable clothing – and you can increase your energy levels, manage your stress, and prevent a number of ailments. Chi kung is said to improve concentration and even increase creativity and inspiration.

The breath, movement, and postures it uses all have specific effects on the production and circulation of the lymph. They work in various ways – by contracting the muscles of the body, by using gravity (certain postures invert the limbs), and by deep breathing, which pumps the lymph very effectively and also fully oxygenates the blood.

The beauty of chi kung is that absolutely anyone can do it: if you are too weak to stand, there are sitting exercises. And if you can't even sit, there are lying down exercises!

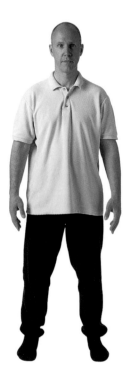

THE STARTING POSITION

This is the basic posture of chi kung. It puts you in the correct position and helps you become aware of your entire body.

1 *Stand with your feet shoulder-width apart. Find your natural balance – your weight should neither be too far forwards or too far back or it will cause tension and tiredness.*

2 *Feel the rim of your foot, heel, little toe, and big toe relaxed on the ground.*

3 *Keep your knees relaxed. Check your knees are exactly over your feet.*

4 *Relax your lower back. Relax your stomach and buttocks.*

5 *Let your chest become hollow. Relax and slightly round your shoulders.*

6 *Imagine you have a pigtail on top of your head which is tied to a rafter on the roof. Let your head float lightly and freely. Relax your tongue, mouth, and jaw.*

7 *Stay in this position for a few moments with your hands hanging loosely by your sides.*

8 *Take your mind through the five elements. Earth (imagine the feeling of weight and rootedness); Water (looseness and fluidity); Air (lightness and transparency); Fire (sparkle – remember this should be fun!); and Space (envisage the space within each joint, muscle, breath, and mind).*

9 *Throughout your chi kung practice, keep bringing your mind gently back to your posture – this keeps the mind restful.*

SUPPORTING THE SKY

This exercise is excellent for the lungs and breathing - when performed first thing in the morning it empties the lungs after sleeping. It may also help sufferers of backache and repetitive strain injury (RSI).

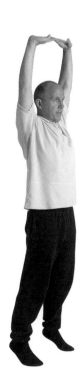

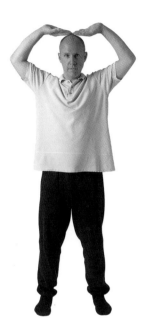

2 ‹ *Once your hands rise above your head, turn the palms upwards to face the sky, point the fingers towards each other, and rest them gently on your crown.*

1 ⌃ *Stand in the Starting Position. Raise your arms slowly and together towards your head, breathing in as you do so.*

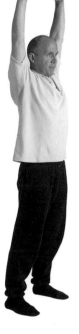

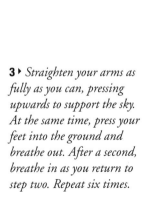

3 ‹ *Straighten your arms as fully as you can, pressing upwards to support the sky. At the same time, press your feet into the ground and breathe out. After a second, breathe in as you return to step two. Repeat six times.*

4 ‹ *Once you have mastered the combined stretching and breathing cycle of steps two and three, repeat it but this time rise up slowly on your toes instead of pressing your feet into the ground. In this way, you will extend your arms and legs fully and simultaneously.*

l trampoline (known as a rebounder)
tive way to stimulate the lymph and
nd health. Rebounding can relieve
tension, increase energy and vitality, lower cholesterol
levels, increase resistance to disease, and improve
circulation and respiration. Bouncers find they shift into
their ideal weight and streamline their bodies – it can even
help banish the bane of cellulite. Balance, coordination,
and stamina all improve.

It's not just wishful thinking: a study in New Zealand
found that rebounding improved resting heart rate in 91
per cent of participants and blood pressure in 50 per cent
of participants. Even more interesting were the less
quantifiable benefits: improved ability to handle stress,
increased feelings of wellbeing, more energy, as well as
greater resistance to colds and flu.

Many of these bouncing benefits come about because
bouncing is, without doubt, one of the very best ways of
stimulating the lymphatic system and sluicing away toxins.
It's the perfect workout for your lymph. The up and down
movement provides an acceleration-deceleration effect
which in turn changes the force of gravity in your body.
This puts the lymphatic and blood circulation systems
under intense rhythmic pressure which stimulates the
dumping of wastes from all the cells.

Best of all rebounding is fun. For those of you who hate
the idea of exercising in public – or hate the very idea of
exercising at all – get a rebounder. Put on some music (or
if you're a TV addict put your rebounder in front of the
set) and just bounce. You'll probably be surprised at how
quickly you find yourself out of breath – bouncing is
tougher than it looks.

But at the end of a session you should feel incredible –
bounding with energy while every muscle in your body
feels stretched and toned. It also affects the mind and
spirit. Symbolically, when we bounce we are literally lifting
ourselves, rising above our problems. Bouncing connects
you with a childlike sense of fun – it can energize and
revitalize your whole being.

NOTES & CAUTIONS

Rebounding is a remarkably safe form of exercise. However, check with your medical practitioner if you suffer one of the following: heart disease, dizziness, osteoporosis, chest pains, arthritis or joint pain, prolapsed uterus, detached retina, phlebitis, or any other serious health concern. Don't bounce on a full stomach; when suffering from colds or viruses; or when you're overly tired.

At first you may experience a slight feeling of nausea – this is natural. Other side effects – headaches, rashes, discharge, runny nose, changes in bowel movement – are signs that your body is cleansing itself.

Wear loose and comfortable clothing. Bare feet are best but don't wear slippery shoes, socks, or tights.

BOUNCE ROUTINE – WARM-UP AND STRETCH

▸ *Step onto your rebounder and stand in the middle of the mat with your toes hip-width apart and facing forward. Aim for a posture like the chi kung Starting Position (see p. 42): knees slightly bent, shoulders relaxed, looking forwards with chin tucked in. Imagine a string gently attaches you to the ceiling. Feel balanced and at ease. Breathe deeply in a relaxed manner.*

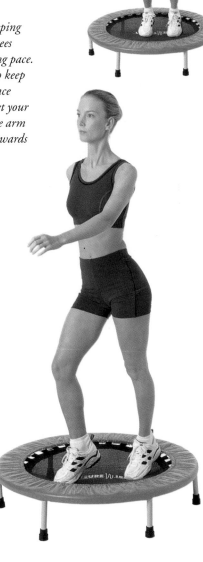

◂ *Gently start to bounce, keeping your feet on the mat and knees relaxed. Start a light walking pace. It may feel strange but try to keep it smooth and rhythmic. Once your feet are moving well, let your arms gently swing – opposite arm to leg (ie left arm swings forwards as your right heel rises).*

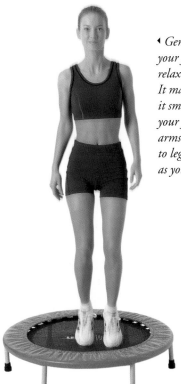

▸ *Once you are feeling warm (allow yourself five minutes) you should follow a stretch routine (see pp. 34-37) before proceeding to the aerobic workout on pages 46-47.*

AEROBIC WORKOUT

To turn your rebounding session into an aerobic workout you will need to incorporate some high intensity moves. Start off with around five minutes if you are new to exercising. If you are an experienced exerciser you could start with 10 minutes and work up. The ideal is at least 30 minutes of solid aerobic conditioning.

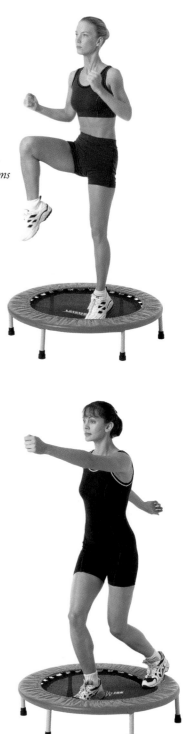

‣ KNEE LIFTS
Raise alternate knees to the front, pointing your toes. Bring your arms from above your head down over the raised knee.

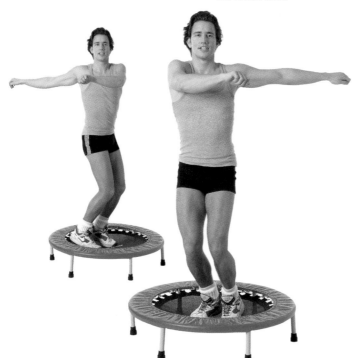

▲ TWISTER
Keeping your feet firmly on the mat, take little twisting jumps, moving your hips and arms in opposite direction.

‣ SPOTTY DOG
Jump and slide alternate feet forwards and back. Arms are moving opposite arm to leg – your left foot goes forward with your right arm. The move looks like cross-country skiing.

▸ JUMPING JACKS

Small jumps which spread your legs just wider than your hips and then back so your ankles almost touch. As you jump out, move your arms straight up to shoulder level.

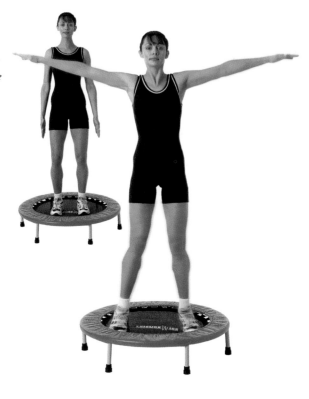

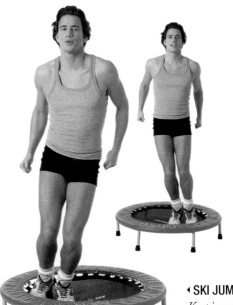

◂ SKI JUMPS

Keeping your ankles together, take little sideways jumps to either side of the mat, as if you were skiing. Your elbows are tucked in and your arms swing backwards and forwards.

▸ JOGGING

Lean your body slightly forwards and take yourself from a walk to a jog. As you get proficient, kick your heels up behind you and swing your arms.

WARM DOWN

- *However tired you feel, don't just stop suddenly. Bring your heartbeat down by walking (as in the warm-up) for about five minutes.*
- *Follow the stretch routine again (see pp. 34-37).*
- *Drink plenty of fresh water.*
- *You may find a warm bath (with skin brushing – see p. 77) better than a shower.*

Which form of exercise would suit you?

Half the battle of exercising is finding a form of fitness you enjoy. If you don't enjoy workouts, you are unlikely to make exercise a part of your everyday life. Spend time thinking about – and trying – various forms of exercise and sport. Is there anything you used to enjoy when you were a child or when you were younger? Are there any sports you have always fancied trying? The following pages offer a few suggestions to get you thinking – and hopefully moving. See Resources (pp. 122-123) for contacts.

WHICH FORM OF EXERCISE WOULD SUIT YOU?			
Exercise	*Benefits*	*Ideal for*	*Disadvantages*
Swimming A superb form of exercise that promotes aerobic training, muscle toning, and endurance. Warm up by walking several widths of the pool in shoulder-deep water and then swim for as long as you can in comfort. Slowly build up to 20 to 40 minutes of non-stop swimming for maximum effectiveness.	Water is 800 times denser than air so it's like working with weights. The buoyancy of the water reduces the weight of the body by 90 per cent, virtually ruling out stress to the joints. The rhythmic motion and pressure of the water on the body make swimming superb for moving the lymph.	Anyone with weak joints who cannot take high impact activities like running or aerobics. Because water is so buoyant swimming is excellent for anyone overweight, physically disabled, or pregnant. And for busy parents – the whole family can enjoy swimming.	To gain any aerobic benefit you do need to be a good swimmer. Heavily chlorinated pools can add back toxins – although the benefits do outweigh the disadvantages.
Circuit training You work alone or in pairs at "stations" around a gym or exercise area. A circuit has two minutes of aerobic work (ie jumping jacks), two minutes of strength work (ie press-ups), then different exercises at the remaining stations. Start with a warm-up and stretch, and end with a cool-down and stretch.	Combines aerobic and strength work for an all-round exercise. If the circuit has been well-planned you should exercise every major muscle group in the body.	Ideal for all levels of fitness – you simply work at your own pace. It often appeals to more experienced exercisers who appreciate the challenge of breaking out of their usual routine.	Circuit classes – particularly the new "army" style – can be intimidating for new exercisers. Make sure your instructor lets you work at your own pace. Warm up and stretch properly to avoid injuries. High impact moves could cause problems for joints.

WHICH FORM OF EXERCISE SUITS YOU?

Exercise	Benefits	Ideal for	Disadvantages
Walking This is the ultimate "no excuses" workout – you can do it anywhere, any time. Gradually build up to walking briskly for 45 minutes three or four times a week (more if possible). Take good long strides and swing your arms.	Reduces high blood pressure and cholesterol. Aids weight loss and may help recovery from heart attacks. As with any exercise, it stimulates the lymph, increases cardiovascular fitness, and improves mood.	Anyone who doesn't have the time or money for "organized" exercise. It's ideal for the unfit, the elderly, and anyone recovering from surgery or heart disease.	If you live in a city or area of high pollution you should wear a mask to avoid breathing in more toxins. Make sure you walk safely – tell someone your route or walk with a partner.
Aerobic classes Find a class to cater for your level of fitness and experience. It should include a warm-up and stretch before a period of aerobic activity and then a cool-down period and final stretch. Many include strength and conditioning work using weights, bands, or bars.	A solid aerobic workout in a safe, controlled environment provides fun and exercise to music with like-minded people. The routines increase coordination and the stretching increases flexibility. Conditioning work will also increase your strength.	Anyone who needs a little extra motivation or who thinks exercise is boring. Generally appeals to women more than men.	High impact aerobics can be hard on knee and ankle joints. You do need a certain amount of coordination to follow routines. Always tell the instructor if you have any injuries, problems, or are pregnant before the class starts.
Weight training Ask the gym or fitness centre's instructor to give you an assessment, a personal training plan, and to check you regularly. Most sessions last for 30 minutes Work out three times a week on alternate days to allow your muscles to recover. Always include a stretch before and after.	Weights allow you to isolate specific muscles and build up strength. Increases your flexibility by fully extending muscles. However, unless you incorporate aerobic activity and move swiftly around the gym you will not be giving yourself any cardiovascular benefits.	Anyone who wants to build strength and tone the body. Training with weights can give a huge boost of confidence as you will start to notice results within weeks and can watch your strength improve.	Gyms or fitness centres can be expensive. You need to find one where you feel comfortable. Not all gyms give enough instruction and supervision so injuries can occur.

WHICH FORM OF EXERCISE WOULD SUIT YOU?

Exercise	Benefits	Ideal for	Disadvantages
Pilates *A gentle system that works by using resistance – from equipment with tensioned springs, your body weight, or gravity. Its flowing, controlled movements and specific breathing patterns improve muscle stamina and coordination. Every movement is carefully monitored to ensure you are using the correct muscles in precisely the correct way. Usually taught in hour-long classes once a week.*	*A safe way to correct postural imbalances and bad habits by increasing the mobility, strength, and elasticity of your muscles. Relieves back problems and is good for toning and streamlining the body. Recommended by physiotherapists and osteopaths, it is excellent as a rehabilitative exercise after injury and can help prevent old injuries recurring.*	*Anyone can benefit but it is particularly useful for people with back problems and is a totally safe form of exercise for use during pregnancy.*	*Although Pilates is becoming increasingly popular there are relatively few teachers – particularly outside major cities.*
Cycling *Takes you into the open air – and ideally the countryside. In bad weather, use a static bike in a gym – those with moving handlebars give your upper body a workout, too. Build up slowly and aim for continuous cycling for at least 30 minutes to get an aerobic workout.*	*An ideal form of aerobic exercise which also tones the lower body. A simple and effective way to build up cardiovascular fitness and endurance.*	*Almost anyone. Those using a static bike can build up the length and difficulty of a workout very gradually and so can watch their progress. If you live relatively near your work, cycling gives you a workout – and saves fares and fuel.*	*Cycling in polluted urban areas increases your toxic overload – so wear a mask. Cycling in crowded streets may make it hard to keep up your heart rate. Use of a normal bike does not exercise your upper body.*
Tai chi *An ancient exercise system that involves performing a series of graceful fluid moves which look simple but are, in fact, incredibly challenging. Classes usually last about an hour once a week. Practice every day for around 20 minutes for the best benefits.*	*Renowned as a stress reliever – it deeply relaxes mind and body while instilling a wonderful surge of energy and vitality. It bestows flexibility, improves balance and coordination, strengthens the heart, and increases lung capacity.*	*No age or health barriers – it can be learned by young and elderly alike. Superb for anyone wanting to strengthen their bones – even those with severe osteoporosis or arthritis. Particularly suits people drawn to its quiet, slow grace.*	*Takes enormous patience and discipline to learn. You need a teacher – it is hard to learn tai chi from a book or video. The quiet, precise nature of tai chi may irritate some people.*

WHICH FORM OF EXERCISE WOULD SUIT YOU?

Exercise	Benefits	Ideal for	Disadvantages
Water aerobics *Like a standard aerobics class, except in the water! Water, or aqua, aerobics is ideally performed in a special pool of uniform depth so you can move easily. You start with a warm-up and move into the aerobic section. The resistance of the water tones and conditions the body, too. Some classes incorporate strength work using floats, mitts, bar bells, or foam tubes.*	*Does not put any strain or stress on joints. The water cushions and protects the body and, providing you warm up properly and follow a sensible regime, there is virtually no risk of injury. Like swimming, working out in the water encourages lymph flow. May also help alleviate depression, including post-natal depression.*	*Anyone new to exercising – aqua aerobics is safe and fun, and you can work at your own pace. Ideal for the elderly, pregnant women, and anyone with joint injuries. Great if you like the idea of working out in water but are not a strong swimmer.*	*You need access to a special pool. Classes need to be well taught to stop you getting cold and bored.*
Dance *There are many dance forms – from ballet to belly dancing; salsa to ballroom; line dancing to flamenco. You can also try "dance therapy" forms, such as Life Dance or Biodanza, which encourage more free-form expression. Most dance is taught in weekly lessons of around an hour.*	*First of all, dancing is great fun! Depending on the dance form you will gain varying degrees of aerobic conditioning and strength building. You will tone your body, improve coordination, and become more flexible. Dancing elevates mood and stimulates oxygenation and lymph circulation.*	*Anyone who likes to exercise in a sociable setting. There are dance classes to suit all ages and abilities so you are bound to find something that appeals. It is also ideal for anyone who dislikes the idea of "formal" exercise.*	*Some dance forms can be tough on your joints. Ensure you warm up and stretch properly. Dance therapy may be confrontational and psychologically challenging.*
Psychocalisthenics® *A series of 23 movement and breathing exercises which affect every muscle group and awaken the entire body. You learn it in five one-hour sessions or two longer sessions. Then you simply practise it once a day for 15 minutes.*	*Encourages lymph drainage, promotes flexibility, and shifts toxins at a deep level. Deep breathing improves oxygenation and exchange of gases. It gives a great dose of energy, can lift depression, and works well as a warm-up for sports or exercises.*	*Anyone who doesn't have time for more lengthy exercises; anyone stuck at home or who travels frequently – you can perform it anywhere and don't need equipment or special clothing.*	*There are relatively few authorized teachers. However, you can learn it from a video – not ideal but better than nothing.*

Chapter Three

Helping your mind detox naturally

Decluttering your life – your home, your workspace, even your mind – works wonders in the battle against toxicity. Managing your time, relaxing, meditating, and acting positively will help you win the war.

If we want to detox our lives, it's not enough to focus solely on the externals – clean food and drink, and a non-toxic environment. We also need to consider our thoughts and emotions, and the energetic state of our surroundings.

Psychoneuroimmunology (PNI) studies the interaction between mind and body, and is increasingly proving that they affect each other. Every thought, mood, and fleeting emotion releases neurochemicals that literally seem to transmit happiness, joy, and peace, or fear, anger, and depression to the body. So our emotions almost certainly play a direct role in our health. For instance, long-term chronic stress can be a key factor in many diseases – from heart disease to ulcers. Equally, research shows that we can combat disease by harnessing the power of our thoughts.

PNI also warns that our thoughts and feelings can be as toxic as pollution and unpleasant additives. If we are suffering high levels of stress, or living constantly with fear, anger, or depression, we are sending potentially damaging messages to our cells.

The very nature of our surroundings affects our moods, emotions, and hence our health and wellbeing. Ancient cultures recognized the presence of vital energy (known to the Chinese as chi), which runs through everything in life. When chi moves smoothly and harmoniously, we find our thoughts and feelings responding positively. So small things (like the clutter in our homes or offices) can have enormous effects on our minds and bodies. We do not exist apart from the things around us. On a vibrational level, we are constantly interconnecting with everyone and everything we encounter.

In this chapter we will be looking at very simple ways to encourage a harmonious flow of chi around us. We will

---

CHI AND PRANA

Ancient healing systems from East to West have aimed to restore a harmonious flow of vital energy in the body. In China they call it chi (or qi); in India prana; in Japan ki, and in the Middle East quwa.

Chi runs through everything – our bodies and minds and in the environment around us, too. Clear harmonious chi keeps our bodies fit, our minds clear, and our spirits high. In the body chi can be directed by the use of pressure (in massage), movement and posture (chi kung, yoga, tai chi), or needles (in acupuncture). In the home and office, chi can be regulated by correctly arranging rooms and furniture – as in feng shui.

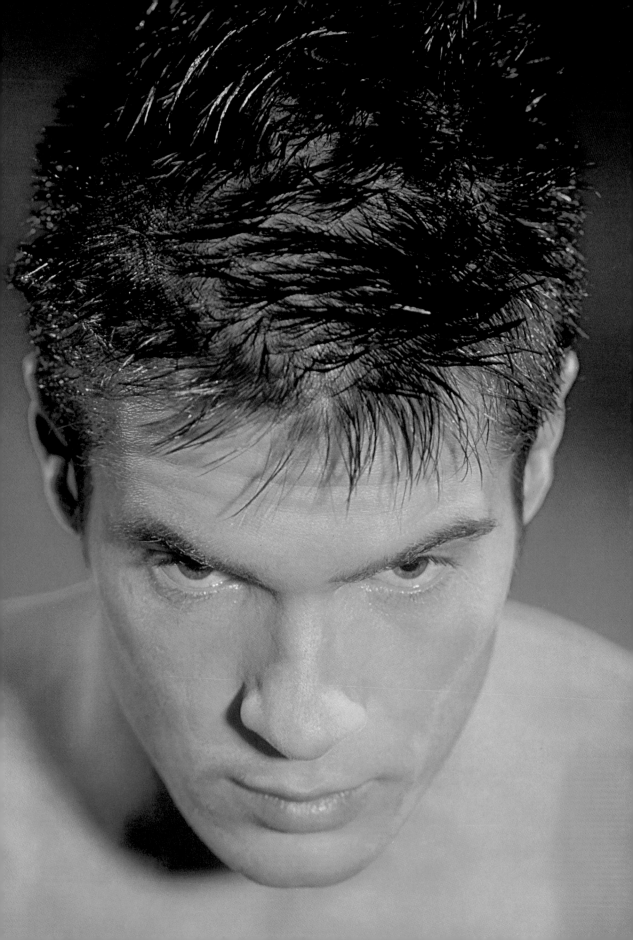

also start to reduce the mental toxicity generated by
a stressful lifestyle. Even something as basic as clearing
your desk can ease the burden on your body and mind.

DECLUTTERING YOUR LIFE

The first step to detoxing your life is to banish clutter. On
a physical level, clutter attracts dust which might give you
allergic reactions. In energetic terms it prevents chi from
circulating freely – the energy stagnates. Psychologists also
believe that when we are surrounded by confusion, our
minds also become confused and anxious. So it is well
worth clearing out the old and unnecessary. The Chinese
believe that when we get rid of the old, it allows the room
for something new to take its place.

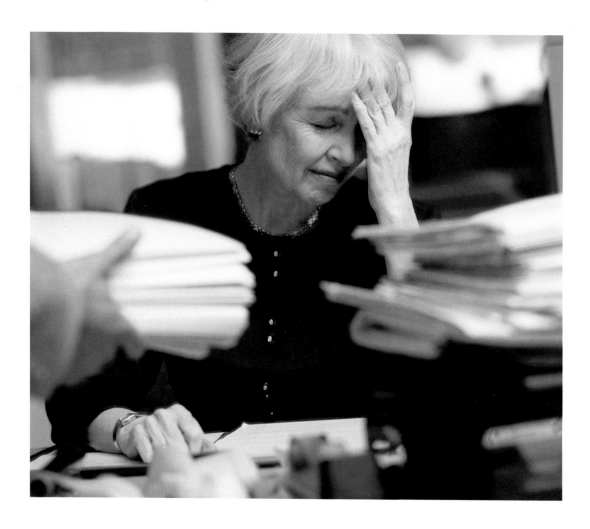

CLEARING CLUTTER EASILY AND EFFECTIVELY

The problem	The solution	Ask yourself	Tell yourself
Closets and cupboards bulging with old clothes that don't fit, aren't worn or need mending.	*Sell clothes to a dress agency or give them to charity, women's shelter, or aid organization.*	*Have I worn it in the last two years? Is it stained or ripped? Does it suit me or fit me?*	*It won't be in fashion again. Either mend and wear it, or get rid of it.*
Magazines and newspapers in piles around the house or office.	*Give magazines to friends or donate to hospitals, etc. Recycle newspapers or make briquettes for your fire.*	*Is there any essential information in here I need to keep? If so, cut it out and paste in a book or file neatly.*	*I can look up old news and find information on the Net or at a library. Fashion magazines are soon out of date.*
Books, records, CDs, and tapes crammed into shelves and cupboards.	*Weed out the dross and sell to second-hand stores or give to charity or other local causes.*	*Will I read it again? Have I listened to it recently? Am I trying to show I have good taste and education?*	*I can borrow it from a library or buy another copy. I am making space for exciting new books and music.*
Letters, papers, bills stuffed in drawers.	*Keep an "essential papers" file, containing important documents. Keep sentimental letters in a beautiful box. Put important contacts in an address book or on disk.*	*Will I need it again? Do I legally need to keep it? Can I find the information again if necessary?*	*I don't need to hold onto the past. I can always find information again if necessary.*
Kitchen clutter: gadgets you never use, unwanted fondue sets, burnt-out saucepans.	*If it's broken, chipped, or cracked, get rid of it. If it's in good condition but you don't use it, advertise it or donate it to charity.*	*Do I use it? Do I like it? Is it chipped or cracked or broken? Do I have too many gadgets or pots and pans?*	*Kitchens should be clean and clear, free of dust and clutter. It's not hygienic to use chipped or cracked crockery.*
A bathroom cabinet full of old medicines, remedies, and cosmetics.	*Keep up-to-date first-aid box, valid prescriptions, and cosmetic essentials. Safely dispose of old medicines.*	*Is it past its sell-by or use-by date? Is it more than a year old? Do I use it or need it?*	*I can always get a fresh prescription. Don't keep medicines "just in case". It's fun to buy the latest make-up colours.*
An expensive mistake you cannot bear to get rid of.	*Try to sell it to get some money back or give to someone who would love it but couldn't afford it.*	*Will I ever use it? Wouldn't I feel easier if it wasn't in the house?*	*You made a mistake: it happens. Get rid of it and forget it.*
A nostalgic family heirloom.	*Give it to another family member or sell it and have a family outing on the proceeds.*	*Would my ancestors really want me to keep something I dislike?*	*I live my own life. If nobody else in the family wants it, why should I look after it?*

Decluttering your bedroom

Let's look at a typical bedroom to see what a difference decluttering can make. Your bedroom should be a refuge of peace; somewhere you can go to unwind and restore yourself – mind, body, and spirit. It should ideally be a clear, serene space in which you can sleep and dream. However, in real life, bedrooms often become clutter corners, a complete nightmare if you are trying to detox your mind and spirit.

Wardrobe bulging with clothes. Check through your clothes and be brutally honest. Ask yourself these questions: Have I worn it in the last two years? Does it fit? Is it stained or torn past repair? Be ruthless and take a pile of clothes to your nearest charity store.

Drawers full of odd bits and pieces: elastic bands, old receipts, tickets, and other general junk. Tip the whole drawer onto a piece of newspaper and be ruthless. Do you really need it? Could you replace it if you did need it in the future?

Bedroom doubles up as a study or workplace. If you can put your computer, filing cabinets, and work paraphernalia in another room, do so. If it's absolutely impossible, then put a large screen around your work area. Unplug the phone or keep the answering machine on outside work hours.

Boxes, cases, old tennis rackets, etc. behind the door and under the bed. In feng shui, the Chinese art of placement, it is considered very unlucky to have clutter, particularly behind doors or under beds. The answer to clutter is not to hide it away but to clear it once and for all.

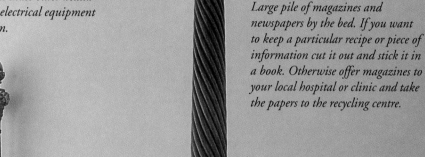

Television and phones in the bedroom. This is not a good idea as electrical appliances emit EMFs which can disturb your sleep and could cause other health problems. Keep all electrical equipment out of your bedroom.

Large pile of magazines and newspapers by the bed. If you want to keep a particular recipe or piece of information cut it out and stick it in a book. Otherwise offer magazines to your local hospital or clinic and take the papers to the recycling centre.

Piles of papers, letters, and photos. Every house should have an "essential papers" file containing insurance policies, mortgage documents, tax details, licences, etc., all neatly filed away. Edit your photos and letters and keep the ones you really love in an attractive box and album.

Dressing table full of cosmetics. Cosmetics should not be kept for ever. Check the use-by date or, if there isn't one, throw away anything you've had for over a year. Dirty laundry in piles. Put everything to be washed away in a basket or laundry bag – and have a regular wash day. If clothes need repairing, do the repairs immediately – or they will sit around for ages.

Decluttering your work space

Many of us spend a large part of our day in our office or work space or at our desks. Keeping your working space clear, clean, and uncluttered can help you work more effectively and lessen stress levels. Let's look at how you could turn your office into an oasis of clarity and serenity.

Make sure you have plenty of healthy plants – particularly if you work on a computer (see p. 24).

Your desk should be as clear as possible. Ideally, keep only what you are actively working with on your desk. This allows your mind to concentrate fully on the task in hand. According to feng shui, you should have a light in the top left hand corner of your desk and a vase of fresh flowers.

Keep your office or work space well-lit, bright, and airy. Ideally you should sit diagonally opposite the door so you can see people coming in. Do not sit with your back to a window. Allow air to circulate by keeping a window slightly open.

Don't allow papers to pile up on the floor around your office – keep everything tidied away. When papers come into the office decide immediately what to do with them: act on them at once, file for future use, or throw them away.

Personalize your office – put an inspirational picture on your desk or on the wall ahead of your desk. Place a favourite crystal on top of your computer.

Boost your chi energy by having a night light or aromatherapy scented candle burning on your desk. Put wind-chimes just behind your office door so they gently tinkle when you enter. A fish tank with goldfish and an aerator provides wonderfully energizing chi.

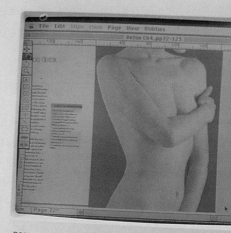

Keep essential papers and documents neatly stored in a filing cabinet or chest. Devote time once a year to going through all your stored material to ensure it is still necessary and still up to date.

Decluttering your mind

If your mind were your home what would you see? A clear calm focused space or a frenetic, messy, disorganized dump? Perhaps it's somewhere in between. But just try pausing for a moment, right now, and not thinking of anything at all for the next five minutes. Impossible? Most likely. You probably can't empty your mind for more than a few seconds before some thought, some idea, some anxious concern breaks through. It just goes to show that our minds can be as cluttered as any room or as any home – and usually are.

It's not surprising: we are living in a world which is changing faster than ever before. Just think: there are people alive who grew up without air travel, without television, without computers, without superstores and convenience foods. This is not to say that they weren't exposed to stressful factors then – certainly life could be excessively hard. Yet the sheer speed of life wasn't there. Nowadays, we are all jugglers – balancing the needs and problems of home and career in ways our ancestors would have been stunned to contemplate.

There's very little peace and quiet in the modern world. We have phones and faxes, voice mail, mobile phones, and pagers. There are papers and magazines; television and radio; e-mail and the Internet. Sometimes it feels like we're all in danger of becoming lost in the information superhighway, speeding the wrong way down the fast lane. There aren't enough hours in the day; you simply don't have enough brain cells... information overload.

Although life feels faster in every way, experts say we are in fact losing time, not gaining it. All too often things accumulate and push us over the top into the burnout zone. We are suffering from stress and stress is a major contributing factor to toxicity.

So a vital part of your detox program is to detox your mind; to clear the clutter and banish information overload. Over the next few pages we'll discuss how to reclaim your mind for yourself.

INFORMATION OVERLOAD

To stop your mind becoming cluttered by too much unnecessary information:

- *Always ask not to be put on mailing lists when replying to advertisements.*
- *Send junk mail back to sender, asking to be removed from their list.*
- *Do not give out your e-mail address to web-sites, unless absolutely necessary – and then insist your address is not put on mailing lists.*
- *Consider cutting down or cutting out the magazines and papers you buy.*
- *Only watch television programs you are really interested in. Then switch off.*
- *Limit your Internet surfing to essential inquiries – or to a certain amount of time.*

QUESTIONNAIRE: HOW TOXIC IS YOUR MIND?

Really think about these questions before you answer them. Take your time. It might help to write down more than a simple yes or no. Take this opportunity to explore your mind and see if mental toxicity is a problem for you. What do your answers tell you? Are you suffering from undue stress? Are your mind and emotions overloaded? If you have said yes to more than a couple of the questions below, the answer may well be yes. Don't panic: pay attention to how you feel. Look at each answer – is this a recent or long-standing issue? On a scale of one to ten, how bad is it?

Many of the symptoms of stress and overload can be relieved enormously when you start detoxing. Exercise, good eating, and breathing can all help to soothe your mind and emotions.

1 Do you have difficulty concentrating? *yes* ☐ *no* ☐

2 Do you often find it hard to make decisions? *yes* ☐ *no* ☐

3 Do you often feel irritable? Do you snap at friends, family, or colleagues? *yes* ☐ *no* ☐

4 Do you worry excessively? Do you always imagine the worse will happen? *yes* ☐ *no* ☐

5 Do you often lose your temper? *yes* ☐ *no* ☐

6 Are you a fearful person? *yes* ☐ *no* ☐

7 Do you express your feelings? *yes* ☐ *no* ☐

8 Do you have low self-esteem, put yourself down, or allow others to? *yes* ☐ *no* ☐

9 Do you envy other people and feel dissatisfied with your own life? *yes* ☐ *no* ☐

10 Do you feel there simply isn't enough time in the day to achieve everything? *yes* ☐ *no* ☐

11 Do you find it hard to sit still and relax? *yes* ☐ *no* ☐

12 Do you regularly find yourself doing more than one thing at a time? *yes* ☐ *no* ☐

13 Do you have to work to deadlines or under pressure? *yes* ☐ *no* ☐

14 Do you have addictive behaviour patterns? *yes* ☐ *no* ☐

15 Do you find you have no time for yourself? Are you always on the go? *yes* ☐ *no* ☐

16 Do you feel resentful of your role in life? *yes* ☐ *no* ☐

17 Do you have trouble sleeping, wake frequently, or suffer from nightmares? *yes* ☐ *no* ☐

18 Do you still feel tired when you wake in the morning? *yes* ☐ *no* ☐

19 Do you often want to cry? *yes* ☐ *no* ☐

20 Do you feel guilty? Do you regularly take the blame? *yes* ☐ *no* ☐

Total ☐☐ ☐☐

Time management

Time is our greatest modern enemy. "If only I had more hours in the day; if only I had time to retrain, to learn that language, to write a book – then life would be great." But it doesn't have to be that way. Time management is the key to ending panic, learning how to run our lives rather than letting our lives run us. It is the key to relieving stress and reducing toxic overload. Follow these simple guidelines to help you put time back on your side.

Identify your priorities

What is important in your life? Really important? Sit down and think about how you want your life to be. List your priorities. Are you spending all your time working and not having any fun with your family? Do you yearn to be creative but can't find the time to pursue your dream? Write down how you envisage a more balanced life.

Set up planning sessions

Once you know what you want to do, you can concentrate on how to do it. Set aside regular times for planning: once a year (for an overview), monthly (for middle-distance), weekly (for closer focus), and daily (for an action plan). In each case, ask yourself what you want to get out of the period ahead. What are your goals, your most important tasks? How much time have you already committed (ie to holidays, courses, family, meetings)? What long-term large projects do you have?

Give yourself five minutes a day

Daily planning will make an instantly noticeable effect on your life. Five minutes at the end of each day preparing for the next could save you hours. You feel in control, which boosts your energy and calms your mind. Putting your subconscious to work will start to produce ideas and solutions – even while you sleep.

Identify tomorrow's regular scheduled tasks and then decide what you would like to achieve. Remember to add in any travelling time. What short one-off tasks (phone calls, letters, birthday cards) can be slotted in to a few spare minutes?. Don't make long lists of everything you have to do – it is demoralizing and causes lack of concentration. Analyze what has priority and plan accordingly. Finally, spend a few minutes getting everything ready.

Keep a sense of balance

It's great to be efficient but don't let it rule your life! In other words don't become a monster, even if you are an efficient monster. Balance is the key and effective time management is about giving you and the people you work with and live with better quality time: it is not about running your life like a Spartan health camp. You can have all the time you need to work effectively, to socialize and play, to work steadily towards fulfiling your goals and still have time to collapse on the sofa on a Sunday afternoon without feeling guilty.

RECLAIMING YOUR LIFE

Time stealers

1 *The telephone. Keep calls short and to the point. Phone people just before lunch and before they finish work – they won't keep you chatting so long! Set aside phone-free periods for tasks that need concentration and bunch all your calls into set phone periods.*

2 *Drop-in visitors. These are the people who say "have you got a minute" and then chat for hours. Make it clear to people when you can be interrupted and when not. Use body language to dissuade persistent pests – stand up and look them straight in the eye rather than sitting in a relaxed open posture.*

3 *Inefficient meetings. What is the meeting for? How long does it need to take? Is it really necessary? Be clear, concise, and set a time limit.*

4 *Disorganization. Lack of planning, lack of priorities, papers all over your desk or table. Keep everything clear, focused, direct, and tidy.*

5 *Inability to say "no". Are you scared of offending people? Do you take on far more than you can logistically cope with? Know how much available time you have, then judge whether you can take on more work. If not, say so clearly and politely.*

Time savers

1 *A clear desk. Keep only one thing, the thing you are actually working on, on your desk.*

2 *Look at each piece of paper as it arrives and make a decision about it. Either deal with it, file it, or throw it away – immediately.*

3 *Schedule "Me" time. If possible allow yourself certain periods each day when you won't be disturbed. Use them for dealing with creative work or ideas, or simply for sitting quietly and refuelling.*

4 *Become proactive rather than reactive. Decide and plan what you will do and when. Treat "appointments" with yourself as if they were with someone else.*

5 *Take stretch breaks every hour. Walk around for a few minutes, returning refreshed and with your concentration replenished.*

6 *Look at your energy. Some of us are early birds, some night owls. When are you most creative, most organized? Schedule your day accordingly. Don't attempt something major when you're half asleep – use the time to make calls, catch up on small tasks.*

Relaxation, meditation, and mindfulness

Meditation and relaxation are powerful allies in your battle against stress and toxic mind patterns. So why aren't we all meditating and relaxing? Maybe because meditation is often seen as something difficult, mystical, and maybe even boring. Maybe because we are so caught up in the frenzy of modern life we feel guilty about taking even a few moments to relax. Yet as little as five or ten minutes a day spent on these exercises could help you to compose yourself and declutter your mind. They are very simple but profoundly effective.

BASIC MEDITATION EXERCISE

1 Sit with an alert and relaxed body posture so you feel comfortable, either in a straight-backed chair with your feet flat on the floor or on a thick firm cushion, 7.5 to 15 centimetres (3 to 6 inches) off the floor.

2 Keep your back straight, aligned with your head and neck, and relax your body.

3 Start to breathe steadily and deeply. Observe the breath as it flows in and out, feeling your stomach falling and rising. Give it your full attention.

4 If you find your attention starts to wander, simply note the fact and gently bring your thoughts back to your breath, to the rising and falling of your stomach.

5 Try to sit for around 20 minutes.

6 Don't jump up immediately afterwards. Bring yourself slowly back to normal consciousness. Become aware of the room around you, gently stretch and "come back" fully before standing up.

There are many different ways of meditating. If this doesn't work for you try these alternatives:

▪ Sit in front of a lighted candle. Gently focus your eyes on the candle flame and watch it. Keep your attention on the flame.

▪ Slowly count from one to ten in your head, keeping your attention on the number. If you feel your attention wandering, go back to one and start again. (Don't worry – few people make anywhere near ten to begin with!).

▪ Choose a mantra, a sacred sound, or favourite word or phrase. Sit comfortably and repeat your chosen phrase.

MUSCLE RELAXATION

A great exercise if you're stressed, tired, tense, or can't sleep.

1 *Lie down in a peaceful room. Be comfortable and warm.*

2 *Take ten deep breaths and gently close your eyes.*

3 *Now take your attention into your head. Tense your head as hard as you can for a few seconds. Then suddenly, let it all go. Your head is relaxed.*

4 *Tense your face – eyelids, cheeks, jaw, mouth – and let go.*

5 *Continue through your whole body – neck, shoulders, arms, and hands. Then your chest, abdomen, hips, buttocks, thighs, knees, calves, feet, and toes.*

6 *Now check through your body. Are you still holding tension anywhere? If so, go back and focus on that part again.*

It might be "Ohm", a vowel sound like "aaaaah", or a phrase like "I am at peace." Choose something which is meaningful to you.

Visualization

Visualization techniques are incredibly effective. If you practise them regularly, you will find that you can put yourself into an instant state of calm anywhere, at any time, simply by recalling the visualization. Imagining yourself in a calm, beautiful place is one of the key strategies suggested by organisations such as the American Institute of Stress. Ideally, you should practise this technique when you are not stressed, for the first few times, so you can build up the relaxed atmosphere. Thereafter, it is a superb stressbuster.

1 Sit or lie in a warm and comfortable place. Gently shut your eyes.

2 Count from one to ten, telling yourself with each number that you are becoming more relaxed as you go deeper and deeper into peace.

3 Think about a place in which you could feel totally comfortable and safe. It might be real or imaginary: perhaps a beautiful beach; a woodland glade; a warm room with a cosy armchair…

4 Start to build up a clear picture of this place in your head. What does it look like? What does it smell like? What sounds can you hear? Can you feel the sand or grass or warm blanket?

5 Practise until you really know your place. Then, having set up your private refuge you can escape into it whenever the stress levels start to rise.

MINDFULNESS – A MODERN MEDITATION

There is another technique which is even more simple than meditation and relaxation. Mindfulness is meditation brought up to date, pared of its mystical and religious connotations, and honed to slot into the most frenetic Western life. It is a clear form of mind-body medicine. The simple idea is to put you back in control of your life, learning how to listen to your mind and body rather than being tossed around by the world outside. It has been

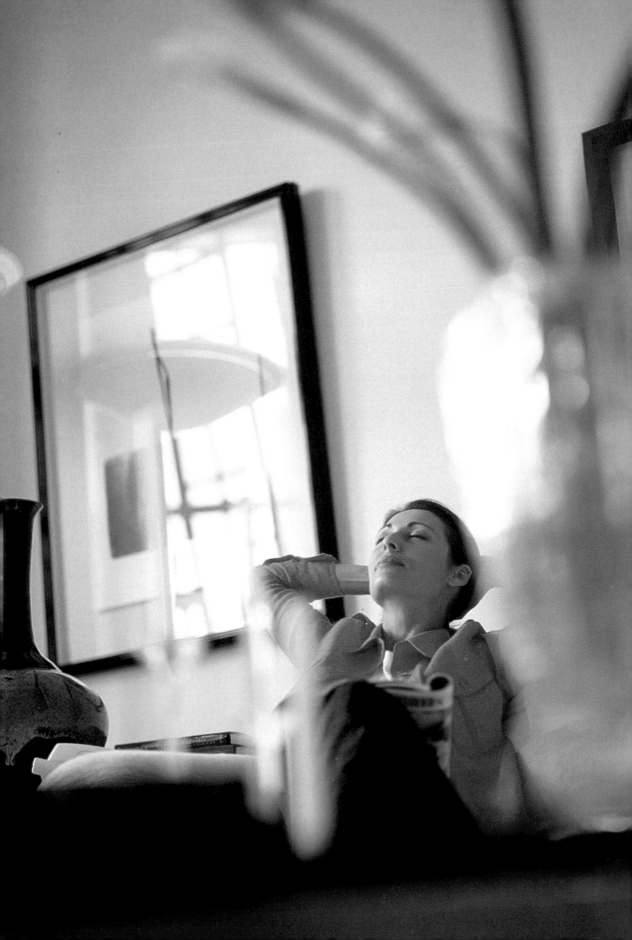

pioneered by Jon Kabat-Zinn of the Stress Reduction Clinic at the University of Massachusetts Hospital who has found that mindfulness can help all manner of problems – from psoriasis to chronic pain. He has instructed patients whose illnesses range from heart disease to ulcerative colitis, from diabetes to cancer. He also finds the technique can lessen feelings of anxiety and depression – ideal for our detox purposes.

It is a simple technique (see below). At its very basic level, mindfulness simply involves stopping and becoming aware of the moment. The easiest way to do it is to focus on your breathing, gently letting go any stray thoughts or worries that emerge. Ideally, you should aim for 45 minutes of mindfulness a day but even a few minutes will make a great difference. Whether it's five minutes or five seconds, just breathe and let go. Give yourself permission to allow this moment to be exactly as it is and allow yourself to be exactly as you are.

MAKING MINDFULNESS WORK FOR YOU

- *Start each day with mindfulness. Wake up a little earlier than usual and before you even move notice your breathing and breathe consciously for a few minutes. Feel your body lying in bed and then straighten it out and stretch. Try to think of the day ahead as an adventure, filled with possibilities. Remember you can never really know what the day will hold.*
- *Try stopping, sitting down, and becoming aware of your breathing once in a while throughout the day. It can be for five minutes or even five seconds. Just breathe and let go, allow yourself to be exactly as you are.*
- *Set aside a time every day to just be: five minutes would be fine; 20 or 30 would be better. Sit and become aware of your breath and every time your mind wanders, simply return to the breath.*
- *Use your mindfulness time to contemplate what you really want from life. Ask yourself questions like,"Who am I?", "Where am I going?", "If I could choose a path now, in which direction would I head?", "What do I truly love?" You don't have to come up with answers, just persist in asking the question.*
- *Try getting down on the floor once a day and stretching your body mindfully, if only for three or four minutes. Stay in touch with your breathing and listen to what your body has to tell you.*
- *Use ordinary occasions to become mindful. When you are in the shower really feel the water on the skin rather than losing yourself in thought. When you eat, really taste your food.*
- *Practise kindness to yourself. As you sit and breathe, invite a sense of self-acceptance and cherishing to arise in your heart. If it starts to go away gently bring it back. Imagine you are being held in the arms of a loving parent, completely accepted and completely loved.*

Dealing with toxic emotions

Look back at your answers to the questionnaire on page 61. Did you identify any toxic emotions – anger, fear, guilt, jealousy, etc? Most of us have some negative behaviour patterns so don't beat yourself up about it; seek to transform it.

For some of us the problems are deep-rooted and go back many years. If the idea of working with emotions feels uncomfortable or threatening, you might consider working with a trained professional – a psychotherapist or counsellor. If you do not like the idea of talking about your emotions, try forms of bodywork such as deep tissue massage and Zero Balancing.

However, many toxic emotions appear simply because we are not able to express our honest needs and desires. We lack the confidence and the self-esteem to stand up for what we want, resulting in anxiety and resentment or inappropriate anger. Often a greater sense of self-awareness and simple techniques can help enormously. So if you are willing and feel able to look at your emotional toxicity, the following exercises could be a useful starting point.

POSITIVE SELF-TALK

We talk to ourselves more or less continuously. And just as what other people say can affect us dramatically, so too can our inner statements, our "self-talk". Unfortunately, most of us use self-talk to tell ourselves what's wrong with us, repeating statements like "I'm stupid", "I sound like a fool", "I'm a complete failure", and other self-defeating phrases. Many of these have their roots way back in the past when we were given a negative message and took it on board. Sadly, the more we repeat something to ourselves, the more our unconscious believes it. Negative self-talk leads to anxiety and depression.

The first step is to become aware of the voices. Listen to what you are saying to yourself. Can you recognize the voice? It might well be a parent, a teacher, a sibling, a childhood friend.

Try dialoguing with the voice, discovering the roots of the negative emotion. You can use a technique from Gestalt therapy in which you position two chairs or cushions. Sit on "your" chair and ask the empty chair your question. Then move to the empty chair and respond, as the negative voice or character from your past. Move from chair to chair as you have a dialogue.

You can also answer back to the voice. Remind yourself of past successes, of times you've done really well, of times you've overcome obstacles, of times you've felt good. Tell yourself you're great, over and over again.

Try affirmations, positive statements which replace the negative self-talk. Take your most toxic emotion and turn it around. So instead of telling yourself "I'm scared of everything" turn it into "I am brave, confident, and in control." Change "I can't help losing my temper" into "I am always in control of my feelings and express them calmly and appropriately" or something similar.

Write out your affirmation twenty times a day for ten days so that it becomes embedded in your unconscious. Say it silently to yourself throughout the day and out loud in front of a mirror. Write it down and put it somewhere you will see it often.

One of the most powerful affirmations is the simple "I love and approve of myself", which helps to build self-esteem.

EXPRESS YOUR FEELINGS

Of course, there are times when it is wise to suppress or hide your true feelings. However, if you continuously stifle your feelings, suppress all displays of anger, hide your fears, and swallow annoyance, it's not healthy. Failing to express emotion can trigger all kinds of health problems, from headaches to cardiovascular difficulties. But how do you learn to express yourself?

Don't simply turn fear into anger by screaming and yelling. The best response is to be assertive, not aggressive.

Be honest and say what you mean: "I'm really scared of that," or "I feel very depressed right now," or "I hate it when you do that." However you express it, the key is not to deny your feelings and not to develop the habit of always hiding them from others. Always be clear about how you feel.

GIVE UP "SHOULD", "OUGHT", AND "MUST"

Anger is the most destructive emotion: its impact on physical and mental health is well documented. But where does anger come from? The simplest answer is that we create anger by placing unnecessary demands on ourselves and others.

Watch how many times you use the words "should", "ought", and "must". Anger always entails a "should" – in other words, "You should have known better!" or "You shouldn't have been so rude!"

Change the language you use and you alter the whole emphasis. To say "I think it would be nice if you did more work around the house" is very different from "You should do more work around the house." Why should anyone do anything? The point is you would appreciate it if certain things were done differently. So give up your shoulds, stop laying them on others, and see what happens to your emotions.

VISUALIZATION

If we want to alter toxic emotions and behaviour, visualization is a powerful tool.

Form an image of how you could feel powerful and in control of a situation that would normally bring out your toxic emotion. Picture yourself responding in a way that would make you proud. Remember a time in your past when you handled such an incident well. What did you do? Could you use that technique again? Think of someone whom you think handles situations well. What would she or he do?

Think of times when you haven't handled a situation well. What would you have liked to have done? Form an image of yourself handling it differently and well. Be precise – what specifically would you have done? Can you incorporate any of that ideal behaviour into future situations?

TONGLEN – A BUDDHIST MEDITATION

Up to now, we've looked at standard psychological ways of handling negative emotions. Our last exercise is far more spiritual in its approach. However, Tonglen is a deceptively powerful way of defusing anger, jealousy, fear, and other negative emotions. It also has a subtle detoxifying effect on the person you meditate on – and both of you benefit.

- Sit comfortably with a straight back.
- Calm your mind by watching your breath for about five minutes. Try counting 21 out breaths.
- Now visualize someone you love dearly in front of you. As you breathe in, breathe into yourself all the pain, upset, and anger they might be feeling.
- As you breathe out, breathe all that is good in you into them. Imagine their pain and suffering becoming transformed inside you into healing light – you are not holding their suffering, merely transforming it.
- Repeat this for around five minutes.
- As you become proficient at this and can begin to feel the healing energy inside you, you can change the person you visualize in front of you. Take it slowly – start with someone you know quite well; then someone you don't know so well. Finally you can work with people you actively dislike or who make you feel angry, scared, jealous, or irritated.

BACH FLOWER REMEDIES TO HEAL THE EMOTIONS

The Bach flower remedies are made from essences of common British plants and flowers, diluted much like homeopathic medicines. They are totally safe and very easy to administer – just a few drops on the tongue or in a drink. Each addresses different emotions and states of mind. These are some of the most useful for toxic emotions:

- **Cherry Plum:** *irrational fears and thoughts*
- **Red Chestnut:** *over-anxiety and fear for others*
- **Gorse:** *hopelessness and pessimism*
- **Impatiens:** *impatience, always in a hurry*
- **Agrimony:** *torturing thoughts hidden behind a cheerful façade*
- **Holly:** *envy, jealousy, hatred*
- **Crab Apple:** *self-disgust and self-loathing*
- **Larch:** *lack of confidence and self-esteem*

- **Pine:** *guilt, self-blame*
- **Willow:** *resentment*
- **Beech:** *intolerance, have to be right*
- **Chicory:** *selfishness, possessiveness*
- **Vervain:** *over-enthusiastic, fanatical*
- **Vine:** *domineering*
- **Mustard:** *depression*
- **Olive:** *exhaustion, "burn-out"*
- **White Chestnut:** *persistent worries*

Chapter Four

Programs to help you detox

It's time to get down to the practical work of detoxing. Follow the one-month program or the five-day weekend program, and develop the habit of deep cleansing and long-term healthy living.

If you have already started following the advice in the earlier chapters, the good news is that you are already well on the path to detoxing. Good food, regular exercise, deep breathing, decluttering, and detoxing your emotions are the major part of the cleansing equation. If, on the other hand, you haven't already started putting any of the advice into practice – don't worry!

The one-month program will naturally introduce you to all the aspects of detoxing – and by the time the month is over you will most probably find many of the techniques have become highly healthy habits. Psychologists say that it takes a full month for any kind of activity to become a habit – so four weeks of deep cleansing and healthy living could become a lifelong choice.

Most people would benefit from starting with the one-month program. Its aim is to kick start the whole cleansing process in a gentle, safe, and sensible way. Few people are able to take a month off while they detox so the program has been designed to fit in with your normal, everyday life – although try to be as gentle on yourself as you can.

Once you have undergone the one-month program, the aim is that you turn to the five-day weekend detox as a regular boost – every three months or whenever you feel it is necessary.

However, if for any reason you cannot commit to the one-month program immediately, it doesn't matter. This is where the weekend detox really comes into its own. It will still give you excellent results – just because it is short, don't underestimate its powers. The weekend detox is designed as a swift "pick-me-up" and also a chance to "stop the world" for a couple of days, focus on your needs, and restore your wellbeing.

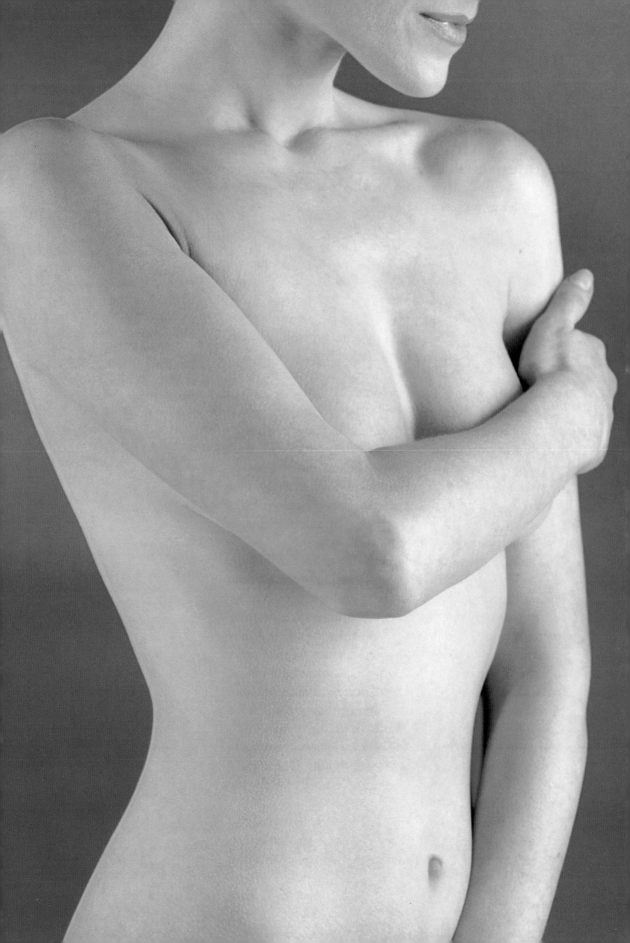

Although short, the weekend detox is a stringent program using deep but safe detoxing methods. Because you will be taking in far less food than usual, you should only plan to carry out this program at a time when you will not need to do anything energetic.

MENTAL AND SPIRITUAL BENEFITS OF DETOX

When you detox you will not only be cleansing your body; you will also be clearing your mind and spirit. While we tend to think of detoxing in purely physical terms, it's worth remembering that, originally, fasting and purification were considered a spiritual practice. Virtually all of the great world religions have, at some point, preached the benefits of cleansing the body as a way of purifying the mind and soul.

Psychologically it makes perfect sense. When you determine on a course of detoxification you are telling your unconscious that it is time to clear out, to cleanse, to purify, to get rid of the dross. The unconscious sees this in symbolic terms, not just as a bodily cleanse, but as a metaphor for a much deeper process. You are signalling that this is a time during which you will start a mental, emotional, and spiritual spring clean as well.

This may sound fanciful but the experience of literally thousands of people undergoing cleansing programs bears it out. When we detox, we start to re-evaluate our whole lives. Often we find that we have been holding onto unwanted patterns of thought or behaviour; sometimes we realize we are living our lives in a way which does not support us and our psychological growth. It is not uncommon for people, while detoxing, to come to quite profound decisions about their life, work, relationships, and spirituality. Generally speaking, people report a wonderful feeling of clarity in their mind and emotions: situations which once seemed impossible suddenly have obvious solutions. Decisions which could not be countenanced before are now taken almost without thought.

You may also find that, alongside a wonderful feeling of energy and cleanliness in the body, you also experience a surge of creativity and productivity while detoxing and in the weeks that follow.

WHAT DETOX CAN HELP

Detox programs may be able to help relieve a whole range of ailments and conditions, including:
- *Headaches, migraine, dizziness, sinusitis, frequent colds and flu, infections.*
- *Obesity, eating disorders, ulcers, gallstones, gout, colitis, irritable bowel syndrome (IBS), constipation.*
- *Acne, eczema, abscesses, asthma, allergies, intolerances.*
- *Arthritis, rheumatism, heart disease, hypertension, cancer, Alzheimer's disease.*
- *Insomnia, depression, PMS, anxiety.*

Detoxing also boosts self-esteem and confidence in
a subtle but powerful way. There is a huge sense of
achievement in successfully completing a detox program.
Often, there is also a deep feeling of love for the body
which can come as quite a surprise if you have spent your
life ignoring or denigrating your body. As it clears and
starts to work at an optimum level, there comes a
realization of the wonder of the human body and often
a desire to treat it better in the future.

Some people even find that detoxing has a deeply
spiritual or mystical element. The focus moves away from
the material and physical planes and on to the higher
chakras – energy centres – of the body: the heart, the
throat, the brow, and the crown. Relationships can
improve; communication becomes clearer; and there
is often a desire for greater spiritual knowledge or a
deepening of a habitual spiritual practice. If you have
never been able to meditate or pray, you may find it
easy, even necessary, during detox.

WHEN NOT TO DETOX

As long as you are fit and healthy, there is nothing to stop
you detoxing at any time of year and you can start either
the one-month or the five-day weekend program at any
juncture. But if you have any doubts, worries, or concerns
about the impact of detoxing on your health, then you
must always consult your doctor.
There are times when it isn't advisable to detox:
- If you are feeling unwell, just getting over an illness, even
if it's only a cold or flu, your body has enough to cope with
and your immune system is under stress. Wait until you
are fully recovered before detoxing.
- If you have any blood glucose problems. These are best
addressed for a period of at least three to four weeks prior
to detoxing.
- If you are pregnant or breastfeeding – your body has
other priorities.
- If you are taking any medication or having treatment for
any condition – whether chronic or acute – you will need
to talk to your doctor or healthcare practitioner before
undertaking a detox program.

The one-month detox program

The one-month program will help to detoxify your body – safely, gently, and effectively. It's not a draconian diet and it doesn't call for impossible recipes or vile potions. It's simple and straightforward, and you will start to feel the benefits within a week (which will make it much easier to continue). Research shows that detoxing can have a significant effect on the biochemistry of your body, allowing the population of favourable bacteria to multiply while numbers of harmful micro-flora reduce. The foods you will be eating are easy for the body to digest and eliminate: they also contain plenty of plant fibre which can help to absorb and remove excess mucus from the colon. You will be helping your lymphatic system move toxins out of the body with skin brushing, gentle exercise, and hydrotherapy so your immune system will be given a chance to get back into fighting form.

Your body won't just become healthier; it will feel better, too. Your energy levels will start to rise and your sleep should become deeper and more restful. Any bloated feelings should go and your digestion should improve enormously. As the detox progresses you may well find old problems start to disappear: headaches, digestive problems, PMS, aches and pains may all diminish or vanish altogether. You may also find your mood improves: detoxing can sometimes even cure depression.

As an added bonus you should find you start to look better too: your skin will become clearer and your hair more lustrous. Your eyes will appear brighter and if your weight is a problem, it should start to balance itself. These side effects are hardly surprising when you consider that you are giving your body the equivalent of a huge spring clean – from the inside out. However, it's worth pointing out that you may find your symptoms worsen before getting better.

Unlike many detox programs, we will also be paying a lot of attention to your mind, emotions, and even your soul. Detoxing at this level gives you a chance to look afresh at your entire life, deciding what works for you and what needs to change. It is deeply transformational.

The next few pages introduce the techniques you will be using throughout your detox.

DEALING WITH SIDE EFFECTS

Detoxing is a deep process that produces side effects, such as:
- *Headaches: drink plenty of water, rest, and put a few drops of lavender oil on your temples.*
- *Unusual bowel movements: if severely constipated, try eating a handful of linseed which has been previosly soaked in water.*
- *Furry tongue: scrape with a toothbrush or a special tongue scraper. Rinse your mouth with lemon juice and water.*
- *Spots, rashes, pimples: let the toxins out and keep skin clean.*
- *Tiredness: make sure you are eating enough.*
- *Bad body odour and breath: skin brush regularly and add essential oils to your bath. Chew parsley for bad breath.*

Skin brushing

First thing in the morning, before you take your bath or shower, you should give yourself at least five minutes of dry skin brushing – using a natural bristle brush with a long handle. Repeat the process again before you take your evening bath. Skin brushing is one of the simplest detox treatments yet it is an extremely effective way of stimulating the lymphatic system and encouraging the expulsion of toxins. The rhythmic brushing can move sluggish lymph and soften any impacted lymph mucus from the nodes. On a purely cosmetic level, it may help to break down cellulite and give the skin a clean healthy glow.

1 Your body should be dry, so always skin brush before bathing or showering.

2 First brush your feet, including the soles. Now brush up your legs, front, and back using smooth long strokes, always moving towards the groin area (where there are major lymph nodes).

3 Next brush over the buttocks and up to the mid-back, moving towards the armpits (another major lymph site).

4 Now brush your arms, moving from your hands up to your armpits. Don't forget the palms of your hands.

5 Move across your shoulders and down the chest towards the heart. Women should avoid brushing their nipples. Brush down the back of the neck.

6 Now brush your abdominal area, avoiding the genitals. Use a circular movement, in a clockwise direction, which helps to stimulate the colon.

7 Be thorough and brush for at least five minutes, until your skin is glowing. Now you can have your shower or, ideally, a bath. Use the hydrotherapy baths given throughout the programs.

Alternatively, add two drops of rosemary oil to the warm water. Relax in the bath and then gradually add cool water until the water becomes quite cold. The change of temperature also stimulates the lymph.

note: *avoid using rosemary oil if pregnant.*

Hydrotherapy

Water is a great healer and a vital part of your detox programs. Naturopathy uses a wide variety of techniques using water, known as hydrotherapy, to assist your body in the detox process.

EPSOM SALTS BATH

Use this bath just before going to bed. Epsom salts induce profound perspiration and so are superlative for sweating out toxins. This bath is also very useful for rheumatic conditions and can help fend off infections, colds, and flu.
caution: *Avoid Epsom salts baths if you have heart trouble, if you are diabetic ,or are feeling tired or weak.*

- *Dissolve about 450g (16oz) of Epsom salts into a warm bath. (Note: you can work up to this amount slowly over a week or two).*
- *Relax for about 20 minutes. Drink a hot herbal tea (peppermint or thyme would be ideal) to increase perspiration and replace lost fluids.*
- *Be careful as you get out of the bath – you may feel light-headed.*
- *Do not rub yourself dry. Wrap up in several large towels and go to bed. Wrap your feet up warmly.*
- *In the morning, or when you wake, sponge yourself down with warm water. Vigorously rub your body dry.*

SAUNAS AND STEAM BATHS

If you have access to a sauna or steam bath (or Turkish bath) take advantage of them during either of the detox programs. Both will help to eliminate toxins through perspiration. They also help to increase circulation and speed up the elimination process. Not everyone feels comfortable in saunas or steam baths – experiment and find out which you prefer and how long you can comfortably take. Be guided by your body.

MINERAL BATHS

Naturopaths use mineral baths, such as Dead Sea baths, as part of the detox process. You may be able to buy preparations from a health store. Mineral baths are best taken before bedtime or when you can wrap up and sleep afterwards.

Simply add the recommended quantity of mineral bath (see instructions on the product) to warm water and relax for at least 20 minutes. Pat yourself dry and wrap up warmly afterwards.

SALT MASSAGE BATH

A massage with salt followed by a bath is a superb detoxifier and is good if you feel yourself going down with a cold or flu. Salt stimulates the body, increases circulation, and deeply cleanses the skin by sloughing off old cells. With cool water it makes an invigorating start to the day.
caution: *Do not use if you have broken skin, high or low blood pressure, or any heart conditions.*

- *Fill your bath with warm water. Sit on the edge of the bath or in a chair nearby.*
- *Pour a handful of sea salt into the palm of your hand and add water until you have a thick paste.*
- *Massage the paste into your body. Use small slow circular movements from the neck and shoulders down to the feet.*
- *Now get into the bath and soak. You can add a further cup or two of sea salt to the water. Relax for about 10 minutes.*

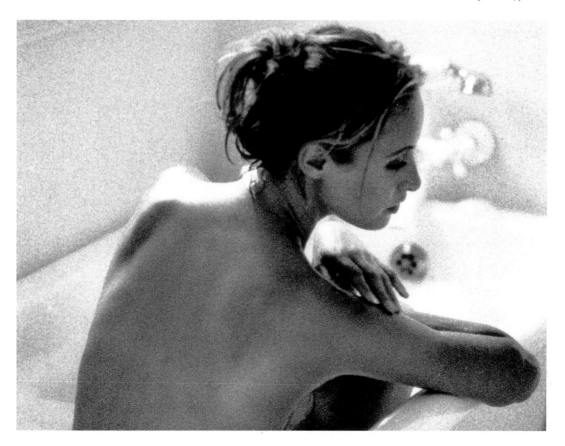

BODY WRAP

Ask a friend to help with this powerful treatment. Body wraps work as a kind of sauna or steam – eliminating toxic waste through sweating.

1 *Place a cotton sheet in cold water so it becomes totally immersed.*
2 *Wring it out, leaving it just damp. It shouldn't drip yet needs to be cold to the touch.*
3 *Spread it over a bed or couch (you may wish to put down a plastic sheet underneath) and lay down on it.*
4 *Place three hot water bottles inside the sheet – one by your feet, one around your waist, and one near your chest.*
5 *Ask your friend to wrap the ends of the sheet firmly around you and the hot water bottles so you are entirely covered – from your neck down to your feet. You are now encased in your own private steam "room".*
6 *Relax like this for at least three hours. You will start to sweat profusely within 10 to 15 minutes but the treatment is very relaxing and most likely you will fall asleep. By the end of the treatment the sheet will be almost dry and may be discolored from the eliminated toxins. You will need to wash it before using it again.*

CIDER VINEGAR BATH

As well as deeply detoxifying, this bath also acts as a wonderful pick-me-up and can soothe itchy skin.

Add two cups of apple cider vinegar to a warm (not hot) bath and simply lay back and relax for about 15 minutes.

Juicing

Freshly made juice is one of your greatest friends in the detox programs – and in everyday life as well. Vegetables and fruits have profound healing properties and are rich in micronutrients. Many of them actively encourage elimination. The majority of vegetables are highly alkaline in their nature and have the ability to bind acids and eliminate them through the kidneys and urine. So juicing is ideal for anyone suffering from rheumatism and arthritis – providing, of course, you avoid citrus fruits which exacerbate the conditions.

THE DETOX JUICES

Throughout the programs you will be drinking the following "super-juices" (liver flush, carrot juice, beetroot juice, and celery juice), which possess the most potent detox properties. Choose fresh organic vegetables – ideally those in season. Use a juicer for most of these recipes and follow the manufacturer's instructions.

You can also drink the juices in your maintenance program – if you feel sluggish, a day on juice could sort out your problems. Many naturopaths say that a day a week on a diet of vegetable juices will be beneficial to anyone, providing you don't suffer from diabetes. Drink around 600ml (1pt) to a litre (1.75pts) of fresh juice – don't swallow it all at once, sip it slowly throughout the day. Also, drink plenty of fresh water – either room temperature or warm.

Liver flush

This is the famous detoxing juice from polarity therapy. It helps to clear the liver, gall-bladder, kidneys, and intestinal tract, and can help restore a correct biochemical balance in the body when combined with a cleansing detox diet.

COMBINED JUICES

The founder of polarity therapy, Randolph Stone, believed these combined juices could help:
- *For constipation: cabbage, spinach, celery, and lemon.*
- *For skin conditions: carrot, beetroot, and celery.*
- *For arthritis: carrot, celery, and cabbage.*
- *For high blood pressure: celery, beetroot, and carrot.*
- *For low blood pressure: carrot, beetroot, and dandelion.*
- *For asthma and catarrh: carrot and radish.*
- *To clear sinuses: mix lemon juice (50g/2oz), horseradish (100g/4oz), 1tsp garlic juice, 1 tbs honey. Take 1 tsp four times a day.*
- *To soothe the nerves: lemon and lime.*
- *For sore throats and colds: lemon, lime, and pineapple.*

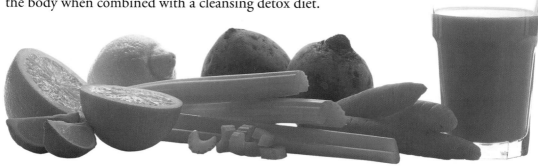

It does taste a little odd but you quickly get used to it!

Combine three to four tablespoons of pure cold-pressed olive or almond oil with twice the amount of fresh lemon juice in a blender. Add three to six cloves of garlic, plus fresh ginger to taste. Blend until frothy.

caution: If you have gall stones or a history of gall stones, seek specialist advice before taking this juice.

Carrot juice

The essential oils in carrots stimulate the circulation of blood in the stomach and intestinal tissues, making carrot juice excellent for improving digestive function – essential for detoxing. Carrot juice is packed full of anti-oxidant vitamins and so fights against the free radicals that cause disease and aging. Carrot juice is said to help balance your weight and to give a beautiful complexion – certainly worth trying.

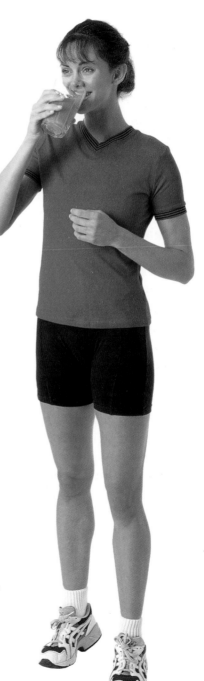

Beetroot juice

The dark purple juice may look unappetizing but don't let its appearance put you off. Beetroots contain betaine which stimulates the function of the liver cells, protecting the liver and bile ducts and encouraging detox. About 100mg of beetroot juice contains 5mg of iron in addition to trace elements which encourage the absorption of iron in the blood.

caution: beetroot juice is high in sugars so needs to be treated with caution by those with diabetes or blood glucose problems – seek expert advice.

Celery juice

Celery is alkaline and encourages elimination, and so is recommended for any diseases or problems connected with an accumulation of wastes and toxins, such as rheumatic and arthritic ailments. It regulates the water balance in the body, is said to help insomnia, and is superb for elderly people. On its own or in combination with other vegetables, it is very helpful in the detox programs.

Aromatherapy

Essential oils are powerful medicines with many healing properties. Several are particularly useful for helping the elimination processes of detoxification. Not only do the oils work deeply on a physiological level but they also have effects on our emotions, moods, spirit, and soul (see chart opposite). The detox programs will be using oils, not just to speed our detoxing, but also to keep our spirits high and to help the release of negative emotions. The following are the ways we will be using the oils in the programs.

Bathing

Run your bath to the right temperature – generally, the water should be pleasantly warm, not boiling hot. Then add three to six drops of essential oil and disperse through the water with your hands. Do not be tempted to use more than six drops of oil. Experiment with combinations of the oils given in the chart to find your ideal blend.

Steam inhalation

Choose one or a blend of oils from the chart. Pour about half a litre (a pint) of very hot water into a heat-proof bowl and add two to four drops of the oil. Place a towel over your head and the bowl to trap the steam. Put your head down towards the bowl to inhale the vapours.

Room scenting

Tailor-made burners have a reservoir in which you place first water and then a few drops of your chosen oil or oils; place a night-light candle underneath to gently heat the water and release the oil. Remember to keep the water topped up or the oil becomes sticky and difficult to remove. Diffusers are usually plugged into the mains and have strips or pads which are soaked with oils: sometimes they are linked with an ionizer.

Massage

Choose a base oil – sweet almond, peach or apricot kernel, or sunflower seed are common choices. Fill a 50ml (2fl.oz) bottle with your chosen base oil and then add between 10 and 20 drops (in total) of your chosen oil or oils. Gently shake to disperse the oils.

SAFETY RULES

- *Buy pure oils from reputable health stores. Check label for added ingredients (there should not be any).*
- *Many oils can be highly toxic if swallowed and some people are allergic to certain oils. So, never use more than the stated amounts, never take them internally, and never put them undiluted on your skin without the advice of a qualified aromatherapist.*
- *Some oils should not be used during pregnancy or by those with health problems – consult a professional.*
- *If you are prone to allergies try a spot test – put a tiny amount of the finished product on your inner arm and leave for 24 hours. If you have an allergic reaction do not use.*

OILS FOR DETOXING

OIL AND USAGE	DETOX EFFECT	EMOTIONAL EFFECT	CONTRAINDICATIONS
Rosemary *Use sparingly (no more than two drops) in baths, massage blends, and steams. Burn it while you are working for a mental boost.*	*Stimulates, tones, and strengthens the liver. Encourages production and flow of bile; helps clear respiratory system.*	*Clears the mind and helps you concentrate.*	*Should not be used by people with epilepsy. Avoid during pregnancy.*
Peppermint *Two drops for a steam to clear your head or use in a burner for a mood lift.*	*A superb digestive aid; helps to tone the stomach, liver, and intestines. Useful if you find you get headaches during detox.*	*Clears the mind. Uplifting, refreshing, and helps concentration.*	*Avoid during pregnancy. Peppermint stimulates the appetite – so if you are hungry while detoxing, leave it out.*
Pine *In a steam to clear the head and lungs if you have any catarrh. In the bath and in massage oils.*	*Stimulates the circulation and helps to clear congestion.*	*Exhilarating, uplifting, and helps confidence.*	*Test before use – pine can cause irritation in some people.*
Juniper *Add it to baths, to steams, massage oils, and to room scent blends throughout your detox.*	*A diuretic which also tones the liver, the urino-genital tract, and skin.*	*Cleanses and clears the mind. Uplifting.*	*Avoid during pregnancy.*
Fennel *In massage blends and in the bath.*	*Soothes digestion and tones the smooth muscle of the intestine. A good diuretic and can shift toxins from the fat under the skin.*	*Motivating, enlivening, and helps confidence.*	*Not to be used by people with epilepsy. Do not use on young children. Avoid during pregnancy.*
Chamomile *In baths, massage blends, and room scents.*	*Soothes and heals the urinary tract, skin, and reproductive organs.*	*Soothes and calms; a wonderful stressbuster.*	*None.*
Lemon *Add to massage blends and baths.*	*Counteracts acidity. Tones the digestive system, the circulation, the liver and pancreas.*	*Uplifting, invigorating, and cheering.*	*Lemon may irritate the skin so use no more than two drops in a bath.*

Dishes for detox

The detox programs involve eating plenty of healthy whole-food – they are not diets and you should not feel deprived on them. These pages offer some suggestions for the kinds of dishes you could eat – but, as long as you follow the guidelines and use only the recommended foods, you can be as imaginative as you like.

◄ KEDGEREE

If you miss a solid cooked breakfast, here's your alternative. Boil half a cup of long grain brown rice until cooked to your taste. Meanwhile grill 110g (4oz) of smoked tofu (cut into small chunks) and hard-boil one organic egg. Put all the ingredients into one pan and mix together well, adding black pepper, a sprinkle of paprika, one teaspoon of olive oil, and a little lemon juice. (NOTE: you can use fish instead of tofu but make sure it doesn't have artificial colouring). If you have to have your kedgeree creamy, add sheep's or goat's yogurt or soy cream to taste.

▲ WHEAT-FREE MUESLI

Mix together the following (choose your own combination) – nuts and dried fruits (chopped), sunflower seeds, sesame seeds, shredded coconut, pumpkin seeds, rolled oats, rice flakes, linseed. Soak your breakfast portion overnight in water. In the morning, add fresh fruit or honey, and soy, goat's, or sheep's milk or yogurt to taste.

▸ WARM FRUIT SALAD

Gently simmer a selection of chopped fruit in a little apple juice until soft. Serve with sheep's or goat's yogurt or soy cream.

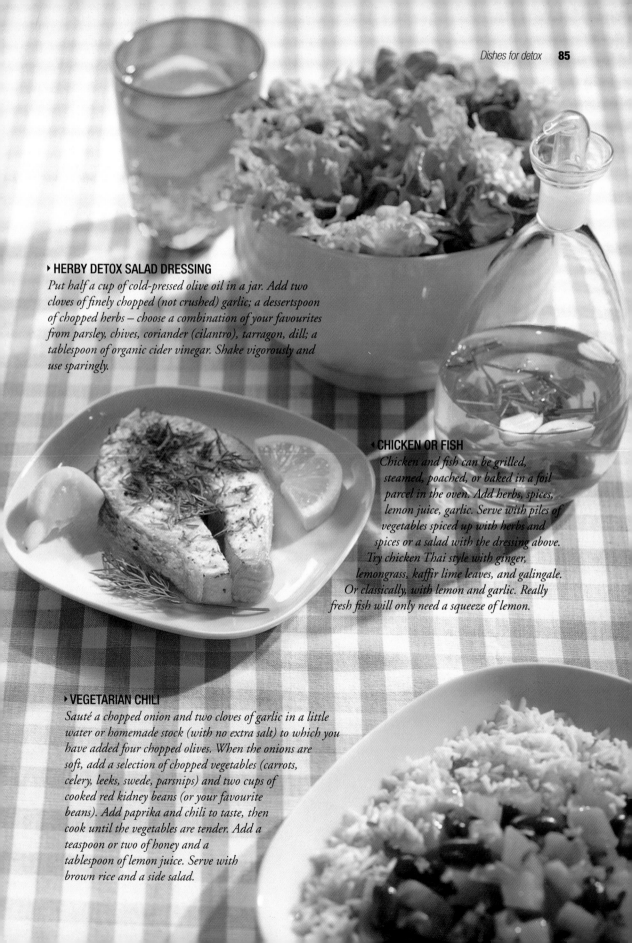

▸ HERBY DETOX SALAD DRESSING

Put half a cup of cold-pressed olive oil in a jar. Add two cloves of finely chopped (not crushed) garlic; a dessertspoon of chopped herbs — choose a combination of your favourites from parsley, chives, coriander (cilantro), tarragon, dill; a tablespoon of organic cider vinegar. Shake vigorously and use sparingly.

◂ CHICKEN OR FISH

Chicken and fish can be grilled, steamed, poached, or baked in a foil parcel in the oven. Add herbs, spices, lemon juice, garlic. Serve with piles of vegetables spiced up with herbs and spices or a salad with the dressing above. Try chicken Thai style with ginger, lemongrass, kaffir lime leaves, and galingale. Or classically, with lemon and garlic. Really fresh fish will only need a squeeze of lemon.

▸ VEGETARIAN CHILI

Sauté a chopped onion and two cloves of garlic in a little water or homemade stock (with no extra salt) to which you have added four chopped olives. When the onions are soft, add a selection of chopped vegetables (carrots, celery, leeks, swede, parsnips) and two cups of cooked red kidney beans (or your favourite beans). Add paprika and chili to taste, then cook until the vegetables are tender. Add a teaspoon or two of honey and a tablespoon of lemon juice. Serve with brown rice and a side salad.

◀ BAKED POTATOES

A filling, satisfying healthy but simple meal. There are endless options for fillings: humus (see below); mixed beans, chopped onions, herbs, and spices; goat's or sheep's cheese with chopped onions and chives; vegetarian chili; tuna mixed with sweetcorn, chopped onions, and half a teaspoon of sesame oil. Add a good-sized salad with a herby detox dressing (see p. 85).

◀ HUMUS

Put a can of chickpeas (garbanzo beans), two cloves of garlic, one tablespoon of tahini, two tablespoons of lemon juice, one teaspoon of paprika, and black pepper to taste in a food processor. Whiz until smooth. You may have to add a little water if the mixture is too thick.

▶ STIR-FRIED VEGETABLES

Heat a teaspoon of olive oil in a wok or non-stick frying pan. Add chopped onions and cook until soft. Add grated garlic and ginger followed by thinly cut vegetables. Keep stirring until the vegetables are cooked but still have some bite. To make this more substantial add thinly cut chicken, strips of fish, or small chunks of tofu.

▼ KICHADI

The great grandparent of our kedgeree, this is Ayurvedic medicine's master-cleanser and balancer. Mix a cup of basmati rice with half a cup of mung beans (split mung dhal) — wash in cold water and drain. Heat a teaspoon of olive oil (or ghee) in a pan until hot. Add half a teaspoon each of fennel, coriander, and cumin seeds. Cook for a minute. Add half a teaspoon each of grated ginger and powdered turmeric. Stir and add the drained rice and beans. Stir again. Add enough water to cover the ingredients with a few inches to spare and bring to the boil. Cover, simmer gently, and stir occasionally — making sure it does not stick or dry out — for about an hour. You can add root vegetables after 20 minutes and leafy vegetables for the last five to ten minutes of cooking.

▸ VEGETABLE SOUP

The variations are endless: try curried parsnip, carrot, and coriander; leek, potato, and onion; thick lentil (any kind of lentil cooked with root vegetables, cabbage, garlic, and herbs); corn and potato chowder (blend the soup and you won't miss the cream). None of these soups requires frying – simply add the ingredients, cover with water, add plenty of spices and herbs. After cooking, blend them for a smooth creamy texture.

▸ OMELETTE

Beat together two eggs with two teaspoons of water, chopped fresh herbs (chives and tarragon are good), and a little ground pepper. Heat a teaspoon of olive oil in a non-stick pan. When hot, add the egg mixture and cook for a few minutes until lightly browned underneath. Put under the grill (broiler) until the top is lightly browned. Serve with a large mixed salad. You can add onions, garlic, and goat's or sheep's cheese. Or chopped peppers, corn, and spring onions (scallions). Or cooked, sliced potato and onion.

Your one-month detox calendar

Before launching into your one-month detox program you will need a little preparation. Read through the detox calendar on pages 90 to 107 to see what to expect. Enlist the help of your family, friends, and colleagues. Explain what the detox entails and that you may be eating and doing different things from usual. If you have any health concerns, however small, talk to your doctor or health practitioner. Try to set aside a month during which you will spend weekends at home and no undue pressures will be imposed on you at work.

Stock up on the storecupboard foods and accessories you need for your detox. However, buy your fruit, vegetables, and fish/meat as freshly as possible.

Obviously, smoking is far from ideal on a detox program – it is exceedingly toxic to your system. However, don't feel you can't detox if you are an addicted smoker. The program will still remove a large amount of toxins from your body and may even give you the impetus to quit. And don't take recreational drugs while on this program. Ideally, avoid over-the-counter medications, too. If you are on medication, check with your doctor before embarking on a detox.

SUPPLEMENTS

Should you take supplements or liver-supporting herbs while on a detox program? Certainly, your body is having to deal with a vastly increased amount of toxins being released from the cells so free radical quenchers and liver supports can be enormously helpful.

However, herbs and supplements should ideally be individually tailored to your special needs. So seek the advice of a professional nutritional therapist, medical herbalist, or naturopath.

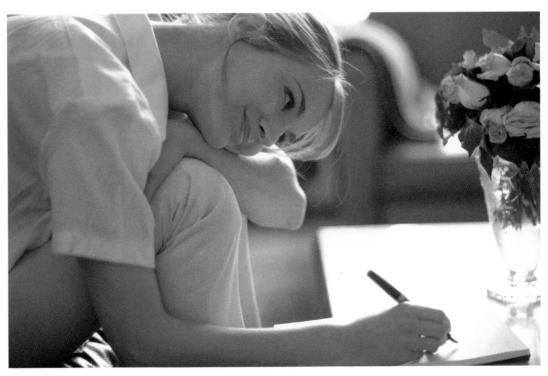

THE DETOX DAY DIARY

Although the detox calendar gives daily variations and suggestions, the basic routine will stay the same from day to day. The following is your fundamental Detox Day Diary for easy reference:

- Lemon juice and hot water on rising.
- Morning stretching, yoga, or tai chi (can be shifted to evening during the week).
- Bath (or shower if preferred on weekdays).
- Breakfast (at weekends, liver flush juice).
- Mid-morning juice (optional during week).
- Ginger tea half hour before lunch (optional during the week).
- Lunch (ideally, largest meal of the day).
- Some form of relaxation – meditation, mindfulness, visualization, etc. Regular hourly de-stress breaks during work time.
- Mid-afternoon juice (optional during week).
- Some form of exercise (at least four times a week, preferably daily). Alternate aerobic exercise with quieter forms such as yoga, tai chi, Pilates.
- Ginger tea half an hour before evening meal.
- Evening meal as early as possible (6pm is ideal).
- Bath or hydrotherapy treatment.
- Bed as early as possible.

SHOPPING LIST

You will need the following basics for stocking your storecupboard:

- *Fresh vegetables and salad.*
- *Fresh fruits. Plenty of lemons.*
- *Wholefood non-wheat muesli (from health stores or make your own, see page 84), brown rice, millet, buckwheat, pulses.*
- *Organic chicken, deep sea fish (optional).*
- *Goat's, sheep's, or soy milk and yogurt (optional).*
- *Nuts, seeds, olives.*
- *Olive oil and sesame oil (cold-pressed).*
- *Herbs and spices; fresh ginger and garlic.*
- *Ingredients for juices (see pp. 80-81).*

- *Mineral water (or water filter).*
- *Good quality multi-vitamin and mineral supplement.*
- *Aromatherapy essential oils (see pp. 82-83).*
- *Sea salt and Epsom salts.*
- *Mineral bath, such as Dead Sea salts (optional).*
- *Cider vinegar.*
- *Candles.*
- *Relaxation and visualization tapes (optional).*
- *Journal for recording thoughts, dreams, etc.*
- *Paper and coloured crayons or paints.*

Week one

YOUR AIMS FOR THIS WEEK

Your main aim is to eliminate all the major toxin-forming substances from your diet. You will be eating normal meals in normal amounts but with slightly different ingredients from usual. Because you will be giving up caffeine, alcohol, and sugar, we start the detox at a weekend so that, by Monday, you should be over any debilitating side effects such as headaches. Start writing your feelings, thoughts, and dreams in a journal. Deal with toxic emotions and thoughts as they surface – don't dismiss them. And avoid deodorants, antiperspirants, and perfumes.

FOOD PLAN

Cut out the following entirely: all forms of caffeine (tea, coffee, chocolate, sodas, and fizzy drinks). Alcoholic drinks. Sweets and sugar. Dairy produce (you can eat goat's, sheep's, or soy milk, cheese, and yogurt in small amounts). Wheat (including bread, pasta, sauces, etc). Red meat. Shellfish. Salt. All ready meals, processed food, fast food, and "junk" food.

You are aiming for a well-balanced wholefood diet. Eat plenty of grains, vegetables, salads, and fruit. You can eat fish, chicken, eggs (in moderation), nuts, pulses, and tofu. Eat as much raw food as you can or stick to healthy forms of cooking: grilling, poaching, steaming. Instead of frying with oil, sauté food with a little stock to which you've added a couple of chopped olives, some garlic, and herbs. You can take a good quality multi-vitamin and mineral supplement every day. As a guide, look out for one that contains at least 7.5mg of zinc.

EXERCISE PLAN

Start exercising regularly. Try out various forms of exercise and decide on the one that suits you and your lifestyle. Read through the hints and ideas in Chapter Two. By the end of the week you should have found one or maybe several kinds of exercise you would like to incorporate into your life – and hopefully tried them out. Practise full deep breathing and other breathing exercises, too.

> **DON'T FORGET...**
>
> - *Stock up on coffee and tea substitutes, and caffeine-free herbal teas.*
> - *Drink two litres (3.5pts) of mineral or filtered water (either hot or cold) each day.*
> - *If energy levels dip, choose snacks such as a banana or apple, a handful of nuts and raisins, or a rice cake with humus.*
> - *If you find it hard to give up salt try adding spices and herbs to your food. Celery has a naturally salty taste so add it to your cooking.*
> - *If you crave sweetness, up your fruit intake or find concentrated fruit spreads with no added sugar.*
> - *Eat three pieces of fruit, or portions of fruit salad, at intervals through the day.*

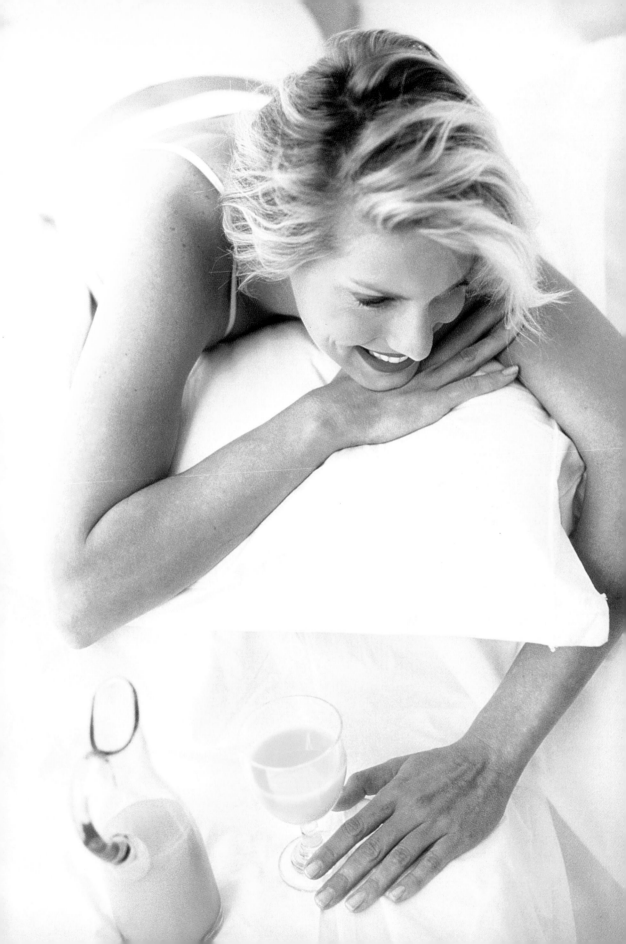

DAY ONE: SATURDAY

▪ First thing in the morning start your detox by squeezing the juice from one lemon and adding it to a mug of hot water. Sip slowly as you think positively about how great you are going to feel as you detox.

▪ Allow yourself time to commit fully to this program. Become aware of your body – how does it feel? Check through every part of your body. How are you feeling emotionally? Excited? Wary? Pay attention to any thoughts or fears you have.

▪ Practise either the stretching routine or the yoga Sun Salute (see pp. 34-37, 40-41). If you're new to exercising take it easy and don't be put off if you can't do as well as you'd like. Practice makes perfect.

▪ Skin brush thoroughly, followed by the rosemary oil bath (see p. 77). Dress in comfortable, loose clothing.

▪ Eat a good breakfast. Look at the suggestions on pages 84-87. Include a piece of fruit or a bowl of fresh fruit salad. Drink a cup of herbal tea to refresh you.

▪ Spend the morning relaxing. You could listen to music, read a good book, or just sit quietly and think. Record your reactions to the detox and the kinds of thoughts and feelings which emerge.

▪ Make sure you drink plenty of water throughout the detox. Aim for two litres (3.5pts) of filtered or mineral water a day.

▪ Half an hour before lunch have a hot drink – ginger tea is ideal. This warms up the stomach and prepares it for digestion.

▪ Prepare your lunch with care and attention – there is evidence that food lovingly and carefully prepared has more "life energy" in it. Lunch should be quite a substantial meal – see pages 84-87 for a few ideas. Try not to drink cold water with your meal – it slows down the digestion. Finish the meal with stewed fruit, rice pudding sweetened with concentrated apple juice, fruit salad, or fresh fruit. Eat your food slowly with mindfulness, paying attention to its taste, texture, smell, and how it feels in your mouth. Give thanks for the food you are eating – think how it will benefit your body.

▪ A short while after lunch take a walk. As you walk, breathe deeply – practise breathing exercises (see pp. 30-33). Become aware of where you are walking and what is around you. Stroll gently or, if you are quite fit, walk at a brisk pace but always with awareness.

▪ How you spend your afternoon is up to you. However, it's worth trying to keep away from large crowds and busy places while you are detoxing. Use the opportunity if you can to spend time with yourself, particularly at the weekends. Be gentle on yourself and think what would make you feel good. Perhaps an afternoon movie? Or a visit to a local Turkish baths for a steam and massage. Or a long lazy afternoon doing nothing? It's up to you.

▪ Eat your evening meal early – around 6pm if you can. Again, drink a cup of ginger tea half an hour beforehand. Make it a light meal – a bowl of hearty soup or a salad or poached fish with steamed vegetables. Eat another piece of fruit.

▪ Take plenty of time for your evening bathing ritual. Prepare your bathroom with candles, soft music, perhaps some aromatherapy oil burning (see pp. 82-83). Run yourself a warm, not hot, bath. As the bath is running, strip off and perform the skin brushing routine. Add a few drops of an essential oil (see pp. 82-83) to your bath. Get in and relax. Now is a good time to use the power of visualization to help you cleanse. Imagine the toxins in your body being loosened by your detoxing. See them in whatever way you like, moving out from your tissues, from the liver, from the kidneys, from those fatty deposits perhaps on your thighs, buttocks, or belly. Imagine them coming out through the skin and floating off into the water and then evaporating into the air. Now visualize a beautiful golden healing energy moving into your body in place of the toxins – it enters every cell of your body, filling you with a feeling of light, peace, and relaxation. Thank your body for working so well with you today.

▪ Aim for an early night. Ideally, you should be in bed and ready for sleep by 10pm. Your bath should have relaxed you and you may well be ready for sleep. If your mind is racing or you feel wide awake try practicing the progressive relaxation exercise on page 64.

DAY TWO: SUNDAY

▪ You may find you are beginning to suffer side effects from not having caffeine. Headaches are quite common; so, too, is a feeling of irritability or lethargy. Be aware of this and take life very easy today. In fact, you should greet any such side effects with pleasure – they are a clear sign of toxins leaving the body.

▪ Follow roughly the same routine as Saturday.

▪ This afternoon, after your walk, try some of the meditation methods explained on pages 64-67. Don't beat yourself up if you find it hard to concentrate – just stick with it as long as you can. You've made a start which is wonderful. If you can, set aside five or ten minutes a day to just sit and meditate (or practise mindfulness) throughout the rest of the detox program.

▪ Keep drinking plenty of water.

▪ Spend some time attending to how you feel. Throughout the program, and particularly in these early days, all kinds of emotions, thoughts, and feelings may arise. Is there a voice which is trying to stop you continuing with your detox? If so, what is it saying? Can you recognize the voice? Try dialoguing with the voice – either write down what comes into your head or act it out. Use the "empty chair" technique on pages 68-69.

▪ Before your bath and your bedtime routine, get everything ready for your first weekday on detox. Spend five or ten minutes planning your day ahead, as in the time management spread on pages 62-63. You may also need to prepare your food for the next day.

DAY THREE: MONDAY

▪ For many of us, it's back to work. On one hand, it can be easier to follow the detox routine at work because you are busier than at weekends; on the other, it may be harder as there can be more temptation and stress can lure you into drinking caffeine or alcohol; or eating the wrong foods (particularly those mid-afternoon cakes, chocolate, or cookies!). Be aware of the potential problems but be quietly confident that you can overcome them with ease.

▪ Your weekday morning routine will need to fit in with your schedule but try to get up early enough to have your hot lemon and water and at least five minutes stretch or yoga. A shower may have to take the place of your weekend bath – but still try to skin brush. If you have time for breakfast, so much the better – follow the guidelines for Saturday or modify them. Alternatively, you could take breakfast with you to eat at work. Fruit salad could be prepared the night before or you could take rice cakes with humus or a sugar-free oat bar. Fruit is the ultimate food to go so there are no excuses for not eating one or two pieces.

- How do you get to work? If you drive or take public transport, keep yourself calm with aromatherapy. Put a few drops of lavender oil on a tissue and sniff from time to time as you drive along. Maybe put some soothing music on the tape deck (this isn't the time to listen to relaxation or visualization tapes though!). Think about introducing some exercise into your journey – walking or cycling to work can give a great start to the day. Use unpleasant parts of the journey to practise mindfulness.
- Remember to take your coffee and tea substitutes with you. Don't be pressurized into having the same as everyone else. Make sure you have plenty of healthy snacks if you know you'll be tempted by sweets or cakes. Also, keep a large bottle of mineral water on your desk – and drink it!
- If you work on a computer take regular screen breaks, at least once an hour. Get up from your chair, stretch, and walk around.
- Eat a good solid lunch. If you eat out, make sure the chef can adapt dishes for you. If you know you can't leave your desk, bring a packed lunch – take-out food such as sandwiches, burgers, pizzas, and tacos just don't fit our detox guidelines.
- After work, investigate exercise choices. Is there a gym or sports centre near your work or home? What do they offer? What appeals to you? Find out if they offer a trial membership or sample sessions. Sign up.
- Eat your evening meal as early as possible – after you return home. If your lunch was not substantial then this will be your main meal. If you have to eat late, make sure the food is easily digestible.
- It's tempting to comfort eat or drink after a tough day at work. Instead, try meditating, practising a visualization, a few gentle yoga postures, or some stretching to throw off the tensions of the day. If you haven't managed to fit in stretching or yoga as part of your morning routine, do squeeze it into the evening. However, don't exercise too vigorously after 9pm or you won't be able to go to sleep.
- How did you feel after your first day detoxing at work? Were there any problems? Write down your thoughts in your journal. Are you feeling particularly tired? It's quite common but check you are eating enough. Remember, you are just restricting the *types* of food you eat not the amount.
- Follow the bath and bedtime routine – but tonight you could try a salt rub and bath.

DAY FOUR: TUESDAY

- Follow the general weekday routine as for Monday.
- In addition, take time to look at your working environment and assess it for toxicity (see p. 25). What could you do to improve it? If you work with a lot of electronic equipment consider bringing in helpful plants (see p. 24) and an ionizer to help detoxify the air.
- Are you starting your fitness regime or new sport today? If not, keep looking for something you could enjoy and fit into your routine.

DAY FIVE: WEDNESDAY

- Follow the general weekday routine as for Monday.
- You're over half way through your first week and by now you should be starting to feel the real benefits of your detox regime. Your body will have thrown off its caffeine addiction and you should be starting to feel far more energetic and also far lighter in your body. It's possible you may have noticed some changes in your bowel movements. If you are looser than usual, don't worry – this is quite normal as you are probably eating far more fruit, vegetables, and fibre than usual.

On the other hand, you may become constipated. Again, this is quite normal. Check you are eating enough fruit, vegetables, and fibre – maybe add more raw vegetables and brown rice to your diet. In addition, you could eat a small handful of organic linseed, soaked beforehand in water.
- If the idea of standard sports or gym routines does not appeal, try to find somewhere you could learn yoga, chi kung, or tai chi.

DAY SIX: THURSDAY

- Follow the general weekday routine as for Monday.
- Think about doing something different in your lunch hour. Is there anywhere you could go for a walk? Or is there a health spa where you could have a steam? Or somewhere you could have an aromatherapy massage (tell your aromatherapist you are detoxing and ask for oils that will help). Try turning your lunch hour into a small oasis in the day.

- Are you craving something sweet? Like thick scrumptious ice cream? Try making banana "ice cream". Freeze whole bananas until solid. Then peel and blend. The result is super thick and creamy – and utterly delicious! In cold weather, go for warm fruit salads – simply simmer whatever you fancy such as apples, pears, chopped dates, and figs with cinnamon and a little honey. Top it with soy "cream" or goat's or sheep's yogurt.

DAY SEVEN: FRIDAY

- Follow the general weekday routine as for Monday.
- Today, consider the amount of stress you take on during the working week. Do you feel irritable or angry? If so, look at the techniques for dealing with anger on pages 70-71. Or does your stress manifest in physical symptoms: tense neck and shoulders, headaches, clenched jaw? If so, do a few minutes stretching in your hourly breaks (now hopefully a habit!). Tense up your shoulders as high as you can in an exaggerated shrug; then let them go completely. Tense your jaw as tightly as possible; then let go. Shake out your whole

body. Flop from the waist down towards the ground – just hang there, as far as you can. Imagine all the tension dripping from your fingertips into the ground.
- Treat yourself to something nice – it's Friday evening! Why not go to the movies or dancing (but stay firm on the abstinence). Buy a new book, tape, or CD for the weekend; rent some videos. If there's a juice bar near you, try some of the most delicious and outrageous blends (but no sugar!). Stock up on what you need for the weekend ahead. Buy yourself flowers; scented candles, too.

Week two

YOUR AIMS FOR THIS WEEK

This week we go further into the detox. At the weekend we will be following a deeper cleansing routine. Don't panic – you have been gently preparing your body for this so you shouldn't have too many problems. After the weekend you will go back to the general weekday food routine, just as you did in week one. We will also start to introduce some techniques to help rid your body of the toxins it is shedding.

FOOD GUIDELINES

- Over the weekend you will be eating a quite restricted diet – but plenty of it!
- During the week you will be following much the same diet as last week but introducing juicing.
- Try to include more raw vegetables in your diet.
- Make a real effort to eat well and heartily during workday lunch times.

EXERCISE GUIDELINES

- You will have started your exercise regime by now. Aim for at least three or four sessions a week – daily if possible.
- It needn't be hard workouts every day. You could alternate aerobics with yoga; swimming with tai chi. Make time each day for stretching.
- Do not take vigorous exercise over the weekend.

TIPS

- As you move into this stage of the detox you may experience resistance from within yourself and a consequent desire to stop. This is natural and we will look at ways of dealing with it.
- Be very gentle on yourself and take extra effort to plan small treats.
- Do not drive over this weekend.

DAY EIGHT: SATURDAY

- Wake up and feel your body lying in your bed. Be aware of every part from your toes to your scalp. Feel your body's pressure on the bed. Switch to your mind – how do you feel about this weekend?
- Slowly stretch your whole body. Make yourself tall – stretch out of your waist, point your toes, and stretch your hands over your head. You may prefer to lie on the floor for this. Take your arms out to the sides and feel the stretch along your upper arms. Bring your knees up to your chest and let them fall over to one side, while your arms fall to the opposite side. Just lie there feeling your spine stretch. Now reverse the position, letting your legs fall to the opposite side. Slowly get up.
- Move into the Sun Salute or the chi kung exercise on pages 38-43 to boost your energy.
- Give yourself the salt massage bath (see p. 78) or your favourite aromatherapy bath. Lie in the water and think about how you will spend the day. Decide to turn this weekend into a serious pampering zone. Fill your home with uplifting aromatherapy scents. Burn candles and let gentle music float through your space.
- Breakfast over the weekend is the liver flush (see p. 80). Prepare a herbal tea from equal amounts of licorice root, anise or fennel, peppermint, and fenugreek. Add fresh ginger, lemon juice, and honey to taste. Drink this during the day whenever you want a hot drink. And keep drinking water, too – your usual two litres (3.5pts).
- Mid-morning, drink 225ml (0.5pts) or more of fresh vegetable juice made from cabbage, lettuce, carrots, and beet. Add radish or onion, plus ginger, lemon, honey, and garlic to taste.
- Half an hour before lunch have a cup of the herbal tea – or ginger tea, if you prefer.
- For lunch eat alkaline vegetables – either fresh in a big salad or lightly steamed with ginger. Choose from lettuce, cabbage, grated carrots, radishes, cucumber, tomato, onions, and sprouts. Add a little dressing of almond, olive, or sesame oil with lemon, garlic, or onion. Add fruit (apple, pear, grapes, melon, or papaya, etc. but not citrus) to finish.
- Spend time quietly with yourself. Read the books for which you normally never have time. Maybe spiritual, mystical, or self-development titles.
- Alternatively, you might consider exploring your psyche with paint or crayons. You don't need to be an artist – think of it as art therapy. Simply take a piece of paper and crayons or paints. Look at the paper – do you feel an inclination to make a particular image? If not, take up your brush or crayon, choose a colour which appeals, and just make marks on the paper. Do whatever you like. Keep going and then look at it. What does it say to you? Does it resonate with how you feel about your life. Look closely – can you imagine any figures or images within your markings? Try teasing them out – do they remind you of anything? Just enjoy playing with colour and images.
- Mid-afternoon, drink another glass of vegetable juice.
- Drink some herbal tea half an hour before dinner. Try to take your weekend evening meal around 6pm. Eat just fruit from the lunch-time list. If you're very hungry, repeat the lunch-time salad.
- Enjoy a soothing aromatherapy bath and get to bed early – you may well feel tired as this is quite a rigorous detox day. Keep your journal by your bed.

DAY NINE: SUNDAY

- Did you dream in the night? Lie in bed and try to remember your dreams and write them down in your journal. From now on, record all your dreams for they are a real gift from your unconscious. Don't rigorously analyze them but do pay attention to them. What is the feeling of a dream? Is it something you recognize in waking life? Are your dreams threatening? What or who is threatening you? Try dialoguing with these characters as you have already done with your inner "voices". Or try painting the dream.
- Follow the same basic routine as yesterday. Make time for some gentle exercise. Take the chance to walk somewhere natural.

Investigate tai chi or chi kung, if you haven't already. Practise a relaxation technique.

- Make your evening meal larger than Saturday's – eat plenty of steamed vegetables and a solid portion of brown rice. Follow up with fruit. You need extra energy so you don't feel exhausted on Monday.
- Before bedtime, enjoy an Epsom salts bath (see p. 78) to help rid you of the many toxins loosened during this intensive weekend. Go straight to bed. If you can't take the Epsom salts bath, enjoy an aromatherapy or a mineral-rich bath.

DAY TEN: MONDAY

- Back to work and to the same routine as working week one. Eat a hearty breakfast today as you have lived on a very restricted diet over the weekend.
- If you enjoyed the detox tea you drank over the weekend, keep it up. Remember, too, to keep drinking water.
- Take it easy today. You may not want to go back to the full diet as you're feeling so clean and light, so modify it – cut out meat or the goat's or sheep's produce but make sure you are still eating enough and getting a decent amount of carbohydrate and protein. While you are carrying out everyday work you need

to keep up your energy levels by eating enough calories.

- Take some time to look at the feng shui of your workplace. Do you have your back to a door or window? Is there any way you can shift so you can have a clear view of the door? Start decluttering your desk or work space (see pp. 58-59).
- Are you still exercising? How is it going? By now you should be finding it a little easier. Keep with it – by making exercise a regular part of your life, you will be giving your health and emotional wellbeing one of the biggest boosts possible.

DAY ELEVEN: TUESDAY

- From now on, if you are feeling energetic and clear-headed, you can substitute fresh juice for one of your meals, but sip it slowly. If at any time you feel weak, check your food intake. You may need to include more carbohydrate (rice and other grains, potato, rye bread, etc.) or protein (fish, chicken, soy products, goat's or sheep's cheese, etc.).
- How are your colleagues reacting to your detox? Are they helpful or do they try to coax

you to break the program? Think about how you get on with them. Do you have a "work" persona, a role you slip into when you get to work? Does it vary according to whom you're dealing with? Is there anything you'd like to change about your working relationships?

- Tonight, have a long soak in a salt bath (see p. 78). Don't rub yourself dry; pat yourself with a towel and go straight to bed. You should have the best night's sleep ever!

DAY TWELVE: WEDNESDAY

▪ Wednesday is the middle of the week and can be a tough day. If you're feeling bored or dispirited, remind yourself how far you've come. You're almost half way through and it would be a shame to backtrack now, surely? But today give yourself something to cheer yourself up. If you're getting bored of the same old diet, spend your lunch-time in a bookstore looking for an inspiring cook book which gives great recipes.

▪ Have you tracked down somewhere locally you could go for a steam or sauna? If you're very lucky you may have Turkish baths near you – indulge! If not, at least find somewhere you can have a regular massage. Massage helps to loosen toxins held deep in the muscle and connective tissue. Best of all is manual lymph drainage (MLD), which is a horrible name for an incredibly delicious massage. As the name suggests, it works deeply on the lymphatic system and has the power to shift toxins like almost nothing else. It feels divine and gives a huge feelgood factor – you even look better after it. If you can't afford professional massage, persuade your partner or a friend to learn massage with you. Then you can trade massages. There are plenty of short courses available.

DAY THIRTEEN: THURSDAY

▪ Are you still following the daily routine fully? It can be all too easy to skip bits and cut corners. Go back to the week one instructions and make sure you're sticking to it – otherwise you just won't get the full benefits.

▪ Are you making time for daily contemplation – meditation, mindfulness, or just sitting with yourself quietly? Don't dismiss this – it is very important for your mind detox. If you still feel uncomfortable with all the suggestions given so far, why not check out Autogenic Training. This is a superb form of deep relaxation and stress control which is used by airline pilots, industry chiefs, and even astronauts! You learn it in groups over an eight-week period and it has deep long-lasting effects if you incorporate it into your life.

▪ Are you also taking time for your breathing exercises? Once you have grasped the basics, you don't need to lie down or sit in a particular position – just practise anywhere. On the bus, walking to work, before you make a phone call…

DAY FOURTEEN: FRIDAY

▪ Are you varying your diet enough? Look into the huge array of tropical or unusual fruits available – if you've never tried them, give your taste-buds a new experience! Eat new vegetables, too – your palate can easily become jaded on a detox regime so it's up to you to be inventive. If you want a new flavour try roasting vegetables with just a drizzle of olive oil – or put them on the barbecue (just don't let them burn).

▪ This lunch-time, find a place to sit outside where you won't be disturbed. Close your eyes and become aware of the world around you. Use your non-visual senses – what can you hear, smell, feel? Whatever you're sitting on, sense it with your whole body. Sense your connection with the earth beneath.

▪ Don't eat a heavy meal tonight. Prepare yourself for a second deep detox weekend.

Week three

YOUR AIMS FOR THIS WEEK

By now you should be well into the routine of your detox.
This weekend we follow a similar pattern to last weekend
but we will be delving deeper into the mind side of the
detox. You'll be looking further at your emotions and also
how you relate to your body.

FOOD GUIDELINES

- As for week two – although you could try the
  modifications given below.
- Keep drinking plenty of water.
- Help your liver and kidneys by drinking carrot and
  beetroot juice and cranberry juice once a day.
- Keep adding plenty of garlic to your food.
- Black grapes can help the liver, too – add these to
  your shopping list and eat as mid-morning or afternoon
  snacks.

EXERCISE GUIDELINES

- Continue with your regular program.
- If you still haven't got into your stride, try asking
  the experts for help. A good gym or fitness centre will
  have instructors who are trained to help find the right
  program for you – and to motivate you to keep at it.
  If your present gym doesn't satisfy you, then it's time to
  find a new one.
- If you're not exercising because you feel uncomfortable in
  front of other people, invest in a rebounder or exercise at
  home. Back up the yoga and chi kung exercises in
  Chapter Two with videos.
- Follow the tips for motivation on page 28.

TIPS

- This is the mid-way point. Congratulate yourself on
  coming this far and commit to finishing the rest of
  the program.
- Take it easy over the weekend and do not drive or
  undergo vigorous exercise.

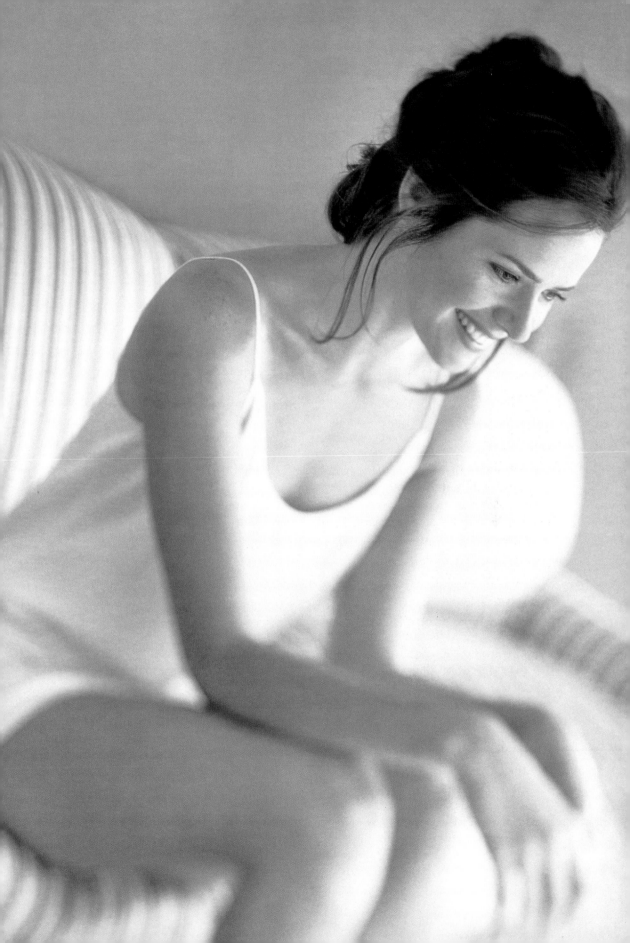

DAY FIFTEEN: SATURDAY

▪ Follow the same guidelines as for last weekend (week two) – so it's back to the liver flush, alkaline vegetables, herbal tea, fruit, and juice. If you are in good health, are feeling fine on the program, and want to go even deeper, you could try a water-only fast or a potassium broth fast today. Here's what you do. On the water-only fast you drink just pure filtered or mineral water. Sip the water very slowly, keeping it in your mouth as long as possible. Drink water at least every two hours. Potassium broth is made simply by adding about four cups of chopped alkaline vegetables to a pan with 3 litres (5pts) of water. Simmer for half an hour – needless to say, don't add salt. Strain the liquid and discard the vegetables.

▪ Sit down in a quiet spot and run an audit of your life. Last week you thought about your work persona. Now think deeper about the various roles you play in life. Write them down. Your list might read something like: accountant, husband, father, son, brother, fisherman, poet, couch potato, cook. Or daughter, student, sister, aunt, grand-daughter, actress, wild woman, waitress, horse rider. Now draw a circle and segment it like an orange. Which role takes the most time in your life? Draw in a segment which represents the time you spend in that role. Do the same for the others. How does your "orange" look? Are you all accountant with no space for father and poet? Are you too much the daughter and not enough the actress? Draw another circle, and insert your ideal breakdown of time for these roles. How could you attend to these abandoned roles?

▪ Do you have an ambition, a goal, something you've always yearned to do? How can you make it happen? Make time – commit to a weekly period of time (half an hour will do) when you pursue your goal. Make an appointment with yourself in your diary and keep to it.

▪ Is there something holding you back from your ideal life? Many of us suffer low self-esteem and lack of confidence, as if held back by old feelings from our past. This detox program may help you feel more positive about yourself. This weekend, read through your journal, look at your paintings, sit quietly, and dialogue with the negative voices. You have the power within you to change.

▪ Sometimes detoxing brings up powerful emotions. Don't try to deal with them all on your own – talk them through with someone you trust.

▪ This evening, instead of your usual bath, give yourself a body wrap (see p. 79) and go straight to bed.

DAY SIXTEEN: SUNDAY

▪ If you fasted yesterday, rejoin the normal program. Don't fast unsupervised for longer than a day.

▪ This morning, give yourself a cider vinegar bath (see p. 79) to help you feel fresh and clean after last night's body wrap, which made you sweat out a large number of toxins (leaving your sheet quite stained).

▪ Try to have a massage today.

▪ This afternoon explore your relationship with your body. Stand naked in front of a full-length mirror. What parts of your body don't you like? Why? Is the inner voice fair to say you're too fat, too thin, too wrinkled, etc. Or is it reacting to old messages or media images? Which parts do you like? Appreciate them and try to feel the same for your whole body, the body that carries and protects you: without it, you wouldn't be alive. Be grateful for your body – as far as you can. Try looking yourself in the eye and saying "I love my body." It will sound false at first but persist.

■ This afternoon, let your body move as it wishes to soft flowing music. Then dance to something rhythmic, with a solid drum beat. Experiment with different kinds of music.

■ This evening, eat a solid meal. If you are feeling weak, add white fish or chicken.
■ Enjoy a soothing aromatherapy bath after skin brushing as usual.

DAY SEVENTEEN: MONDAY

■ Return to the usual weekday routine, eating, and exercise plan from now until Friday. Make sure you are including all the elements. Make sure you are eating enough to keep your energy levels up.
■ Have you fitted any swimming into your program so far? If not, try to get yourself into the water this week. Water aerobics is a wonderful form of exercise – effective and great fun.
■ Tonight, have a mineral salts bath.

DAY EIGHTEEN: TUESDAY

■ Are you having fun? Laughter is as healing as the detox methods we have been using so make sure you get enough fun and laughter in your life. Maybe spend an evening with good friends. Or rent a couple of feelgood movies from the video store.
■ End the day with a salt rub and bath. Wrap yourself up in towels and go to bed.

DAY NINETEEN: WEDNESDAY

■ Continue to use aromatherapy to keep your mood high and your stress down. If you can use an aromatherapy burner at work, so much the better. If not, simply put some of your favourite oil on a tissue – as you did in week one. Whenever you feel stressed or fed up, take it out and have a good long sniff.
■ This evening, relax in a soothing aromatherapy bath. If you haven't been bothering with the candles and music, try it tonight. Practise the visualization technique given in week one. Or imagine you are Aphrodite, the Greek goddess of love and beauty, attended in her bath by her handmaidens (men could be Apollo or whichever god you prefer!). Imagine them telling you how wonderful, beautiful, and healthy you are. Believe them.

DAY TWENTY: THURSDAY

■ Treat yourself to a bunch of flowers for your desk – or a lovely potted plant. Burn a candle in front of you to keep you focused.
■ Buy yourself a small treat – a favourite magazine, some exotic fruit, some new underwear, or a fresh lipstick.
■ Enjoy a cider vinegar bath this evening and go to bed early.

DAY TWENTY ONE: FRIDAY

■ You should be feeling wonderful by now. Luxuriate in this feeling.
■ Go out dancing this evening; go to see a show or a new movie. Or how about ice-skating or bowling? Or if it's light in the evenings, go for a hike or cycle-ride or even try horseriding or canoeing.

Week four

YOUR AIMS FOR THIS WEEK

You're nearly there! If you've got this far, you'll know for yourself just how wonderful you feel on this program. This last week continues the work of the last three – we have another deeper detox at the weekend and then bring ourselves back to normality in the week after.

FOOD GUIDELINES

- As for weeks two and three – although you could try the modifications given below.
- Keep drinking plenty of water.
- Help your liver and kidneys by drinking carrot and beetroot juice and cranberry juice once a day.
- Keep adding plenty of garlic to your food.
- Black grapes can help the liver, too – add these to your shopping list and eat as mid-morning or afternoon snacks.

EXERCISE GUIDELINES

- Continue with your regular program.
- Don't worry if you have only just started with your exercise program because of delays in choosing or finding the right expert to advise you. Better late than never!
- Keep up with your home exercises – rebounding, yoga, tai chi, and chi kung, etc. Have you found a video to help you with any of these?

TIPS

- Don't let anything slide at this point. Keep reminding yourself of the tips for motivation on page 28. There's only a week to go.
- Remember, don't drive while following the weekend program.

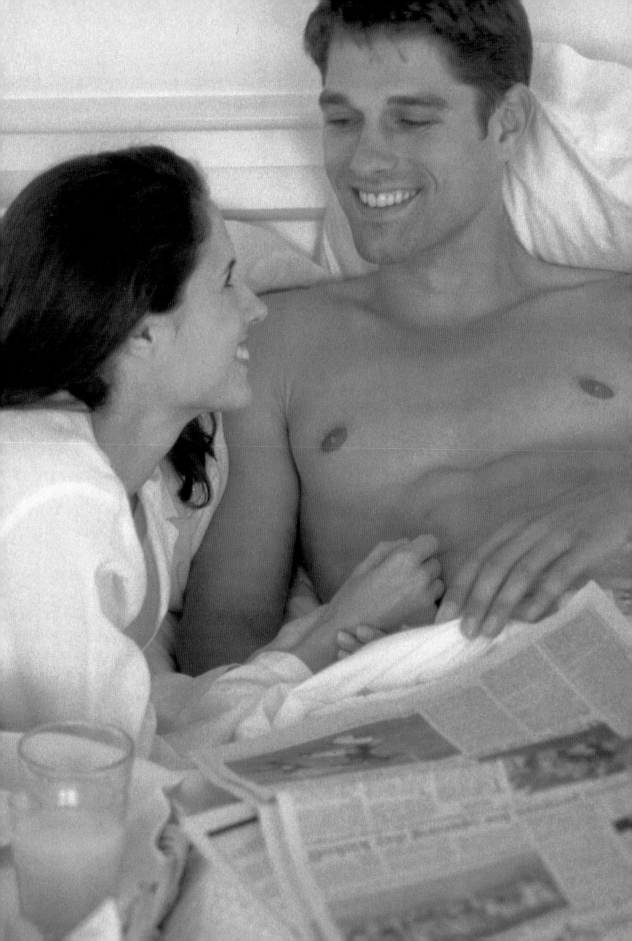

DAY TWENTY TWO: SATURDAY

- Follow the usual weekend plan. It's not a good idea to go for a fast this weekend.
- Spend your spare time this weekend checking the environmental aspects and the feng shui of your home. Most important of all, clear out all the clutter and make your home as clean and clear as possible. You have cleaned out your body and mind so you now need a clean, clear environment as well.
- Give yourself a body wrap this evening. You should be sweating less now and your bedsheet should not be as filthy as before. If this is true, congratulate yourself, you are detoxing very well.

DAY TWENTY THREE: SUNDAY

- Enjoy a refreshing cider vinegar bath or use the rosemary aromatherapy bath on page 77.
- Spend some time thinking about your relationship with spirituality. Do you believe in anything? Do you have a religion, a faith, some feeling of spirituality? If so, does it serve you? Does it give you comfort, peace, inspiration? If not, why do you think that is? If you have no spiritual feelings, do you feel the lack? Perhaps spirituality makes you feel uncomfortable. Why? Put down your thoughts in your journal. Or paint your feelings. Or dance them.
- Try to spend some time outdoors today. Observe nature closely. Watch the animals, trees, flowers, and other people, too. Expand your senses again, as we did on Day Fourteen, and smell, touch, listen. Be aware of your position in this world; your connection with the earth; your part in the whole.

DAY TWENTY FOUR: MONDAY

- Continue with the usual weekday regime. If you haven't been eating animal protein (chicken, fish, game), eggs, or goat's or sheep's cheese and milk, you could start re-introducing them this week if you want.
- Try to have a massage today – ideally, a manual lymph drainage.
- Remember to keep up your exercise program. Think back to how you felt when you started exercising at the beginning of this month – compare it with how you feel now.

There should be a huge difference. Your body should be changing, too – your body fat should be going down and you should be starting to look more toned. In another couple of weeks you will really notice profound differences – so keep it up!

DAY TWENTY FIVE: TUESDAY

- Continue with the usual weekday regime.
- How about a new haircut? You have changed yourself profoundly on the inside. Do you feel like confirming this shift with a change of image on the outside? Flick through magazines and find an image which suits the new, cleansed, empowered you.

DAY TWENTY SIX: WEDNESDAY

- Continue with the usual weekday regime. How would you feel about starting to drink tea and coffee again? You are no longer addicted to the caffeine and so you may decide you can give it up altogether. If not, how about trying decaffeinated tea – and cutting down the amount of cups you drink?
- Why not book yourself in for a facial at lunch-time or after work? Choose a beauty salon which uses natural products. Your skin should be looking great now – give it a final polish. Men don't need to miss out either – many salons now offer facials and beauty treatments for them, too.

DAY TWENTY SEVEN: THURSDAY

- Attend to your hands and feet. How about a manicure and pedicure? Well-tended hands, feet, and nails give a polished look and show you care about every part of your body.
- Read your journal and ask what has changed since the beginning? What have you learned about yourself? Are there any changes you want to make permanent?
- Take another look in the full-length mirror at your naked body tonight. Do you feel any differently towards it now? Do you feel more connected to your body, more in tune?

DAY TWENTY EIGHT: FRIDAY

- You've made it! You have completed a thorough detox program which is a considerable achievement. How does it feel? Exhilarating, satisfying? Or maybe a little frightening or even a bit of a let-down. Record your feelings – try to continue writing your journal (and the dialoguing, dream recording, and painting) as part of your everyday life.
- Try to resist the temptation to go out and eat everything you have missed on your detox. If you intend to return to your old habits (hopefully, you will choose to eat more healthily from now on) ease yourself back – don't give your body a huge shock. If you introduce new foods one at a time you will be able to gauge your body's reaction to them. Some may give you indigestion or raised pulse-rate, headaches, or other reactions – a clear sign that you could be intolerant of them.
- The month-long program need not herald a return to your old ways. Look at managing long-term detox on pages 112-121.

The weekend detox program

The weekend detox is your chance to "stop the world" for a couple of days. It's a remarkably effective way to give your body, mind, and spirit a rejuvenating break. The regime is simple to follow and, because it only involves shifting your lifestyle for a few days, can be an easy introduction to detoxing.

Even this short cleanse has deep-acting effects on your body. By allowing your body to deal only with a relatively light food intake, you give your gastro-intestinal system a rest and help to clear the body of toxic waste. Your body will probably feel lighter and more comfortable. Your mind should benefit as well – you may well feel more mentally alert and find you sleep better or deeper.

You may notice more subtle changes, too. Giving time like this for your body and mind signals that you are starting to care for your true self, body and soul. It can be healing on a profound spiritual level. So pay attention to surprising emotions, thoughts, and feelings that arise during the weekend. Although this is a very safe program, the standard guidelines for detoxing apply. See "When not to detox" on page 75. Remember, if you have any doubts at all, check with your doctor or healthcare professional.

PREPARING FOR YOUR WEEKEND DETOX

Choose a weekend when you don't have much to do. If you can be alone or somewhere peaceful, so much the better. If this isn't possible, explain what you are trying to do to your family or friends and ask them to respect the process. Follow the guidelines on pages 110-111. Make sure you have everything you need before the weekend (see list, right) – you will not want to go out shopping.

MAKING YOUR HOME A RETREAT

Make your home a sensual haven. Buy beautiful flowers or bring in greenery from outdoors. Play gentle music and light candles. Scent the air with aromatherapy room fragrances. Ensure your home meets your physical and emotional needs. If the weather's cold, light a real fire if you can, or wrap yourself in warm blankets; hot water bottles are comforting and help the detoxing, too. If it's hot, wear light cool clothing and use fans.

YOUR DETOX SHOPPING

- *8 litres (14pts) mineral water.*
- *3 lemons.*
- *1kg (2.2lbs) of one type of fresh fruit or vegetable (choose from grapes, apples, or carrots).*
- *Fruit and vegetables for juicing (carrots and apples are essential; you can also include beetroot and celery as optional extras).*
- *Selection of vegetables: cabbage, carrots, radishes, cucumber, onions, sprouts, lettuce, swede, turnips, parsnips. Choose organic vegetables in season.*
- *Selection of fruit – apples, pears, grapes, kiwi fruit, mango, papaya, melon, pomegranate.*
- *Organic brown rice or potatoes.*
- *Garlic and ginger.*
- *Cold-pressed olive oil.*
- *Aromatherapy oils.*
- *Sea salt and Epsom salts.*
- *Candles, flowers, soothing music, inspirational reading.*

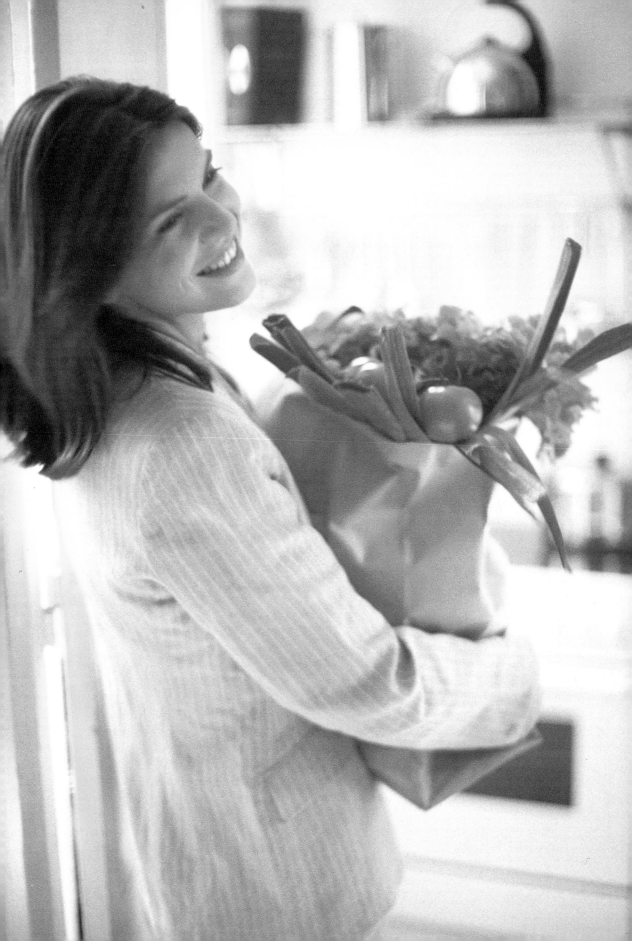

DAY ONE: THURSDAY

- Start the day with a mug of hot water and freshly squeezed lemon.
- You can eat your usual meals throughout the day but try to keep them light and avoid rich, heavy foods. Avoid alcohol, sweets, cakes, biscuits, and cookies.
- Start drinking mineral water throughout the day – keep a bottle on your desk or near you and aim for two litres (3.5pts).

- Make your preparations for the weekend: buy in supplies; explain to friends and family that you are taking a weekend off and won't be in contact; make sure all chores are done to enable you to have a free weekend
- In the evening practise skin brushing (see p. 77). Enjoy an aromatherapy bath with your choice of oil (see pp. 82-83).

DAY TWO: FRIDAY

- Drink a mug of hot water and freshly squeezed lemon on rising.
- Eat a light diet today. Cut out heavy proteins such as meat, cheese, eggs, and milk; plus nuts, which are high in fat. If you drink tea or coffee you can continue up until the end of your working day, but cut down your intake. As yesterday, drink two litres (3.5pts) of mineral water.
- Avoid salt and sugar. Choose fruit instead of cakes and cookies.
- Breakfast could be toast with fruit spread; fruit compote; stewed fruit; fruit salad; oatmeal porridge made with water and served with a little maple syrup and soy milk.
- For lunch eat a large salad or steamed vegetables with lean chicken, fish, or tofu.
- Go straight home after work. Change out

of your work clothes into light loose comfortable clothes.
- Prepare yourself a light supper of salad (with a light dressing of olive oil, garlic, lemon, and cider vinegar) or a bowl of vegetable soup. Eat it as early as possible – around 6pm is ideal.
- If you want a hot drink from now on, choose herbal tea (make sure it's caffeine free), ginger tea, or hot water.
- If you have time, start to clear your home of clutter.
- Before bedtime, practise skin brushing. Then give yourself an Epsom salts bath (see p. 78) to kick-start your detox. Pat yourself dry and go straight to bed.

DAY THREE: SATURDAY

- Drink a mug of hot water and freshly squeezed lemon on waking.
- Lie in bed and think about the weekend ahead. What thoughts and emotions come up? Now get in touch with your body – feel yourself lying in the bed. Stretch out your legs and arms. Can you feel tension in certain parts of your body? Become aware of where you hold stress.
- Get up slowly and mindfully. Try the Sun Salute yoga exercise or the chi kung exercise on pages 39-41, 43.

- Run yourself a bath with a few drops of rosemary oil. As the bath fills, practise your skin brushing (see p. 77).
- Lie in the bath and visualize the toxins starting to loosen in your body and floating out into the water where they evaporate into the air. Replace them with a beautiful soft golden healing light that refreshes and rejuvenates every cell of your body.
- Today, you will follow a strict mono-diet, eating just one type of fruit or vegetables. Choose between grapes, apples, or carrots.

Eat small amounts throughout the day – use your normal mealtimes plus snacktimes in the morning, afternoon, and evening. Chew each mouthful very thoroughly. Practise mindfulness as you eat.

- Drink your usual two litres (3.5pts) of water as well (you can drink it warm or hot). This should be your only liquid – although, if you like, you can choose to juice some of your chosen fruit or vegetable.
- Take it very easy today. You may notice side effects (see p. 76) from giving up tea, coffee, and sugar. Don't undertake strenuous exercise but you can go for a gentle walk or practise stretching, yoga, or chi kung (see pp. 34-37, 38-41, 42-43).

- Take time to practise the breathing exercises (see pp. 30-33).
- Completely relax. You might choose to sit and read – but read something inspirational (not a bloodthirsty thriller!). You may like to paint or write in a journal or dialogue with yourself (read through the month-long detox for ideas). But above all, relax. You don't have to do anything. In fact, the less you do the better.
- Get to bed early tonight – you may well feel tired so it should come naturally. Tonight, practise skin brushing and then give yourself a body wrap (see p. 79).

DAY FOUR: SUNDAY

- Drink your usual hot water and lemon on rising.
- Enjoy a warm aromatherapy bath to wash away the residues from your body wrap. Follow a gentle stretching routine or perform the Sun Salute.
- For breakfast eat a fresh fruit salad (if the weather is warm) or warm gently stewed fruit (apples, pears, sultanas/golden raisins) with no added sugar.
- This morning, try practising meditation and relaxation techniques.
- For lunch, eat sliced fruit (apples, pears, peaches, nectarines, grapes, etc.) topped with plain live yogurt.
- Drink your two litres (3.5pts) of water.

- In the afternoon, go for a gentle walk or sit quietly in nature. You can try the awareness exercises on Day Fourteen of the month-long detox. Alternatively, just sit, relax, think, sleep, read…
- Eat your evening meal at around 6pm. Steam a selection of chopped vegetables from the shopping list. You can add herbs, spices, and garlic for seasoning (no salt) and add a little dressing made from a teaspoon of olive oil and lemon juice (with garlic and ginger if liked). If you are feeling very hungry or weak, add a portion of boiled brown rice or a baked potato.
- Skin brush and enjoy a cider vinegar bath before bedtime.

DAY FIVE: MONDAY

- Drink your hot water and lemon juice.
- If you have time, perform the Sun Salute or stretch routine.
- Skin brush and enjoy an aromatherapy bath or a shower.
- Follow the breakfast and lunch guidelines for Friday.

- Continue drinking your two litres (3.5pts) of water.
- After work, you can return to your usual routine. However, consider continuing some of the detox procedures – see Managing long-term detox on pages 112-121.

Managing long-term detox

When you have completed your detox, you will undoubtedly notice the difference in yourself. Think back to how you felt before you detoxed. Look back at your answers to the various questionnaires and remember your old complaints. Once you know how good you can feel, in body, mind, and emotions, you will most probably want to keep that feeling. The good news is that, once you have undergone a thorough detox, it will never be so hard again – providing you give yourself a boost every so often.

Managing long-term detox needs to become a way of life. It doesn't mean sticking to a permanent detox diet but you might like to consider including these factors in your day to day life:
- Can you carry on avoiding caffeine? Once you've detoxed you will have broken your addiction to caffeine in tea, coffee, and sodas. Could you carry on with herbal teas, juice, water, grain substitutes?
- Cut down on processed and "junk" food – make a commitment to eating food as fresh, organic, and natural as possible.
- Limit your intake of red meat, dairy produce, and alcohol. You don't have to give them up – just don't have them every day.
- Consider having one day a week, fortnight, or month on juice (your choice from those on pages 80-81) or choose a mono-fruit day (as we did on the weekend detox). Once you have detoxed you shouldn't experience the side effects and many naturopaths say this is a wonderful way to keep the body healthy.
- Continue to exercise regularly – try making the Sun Salute or chi kung part of your morning routine. Keep up your other exercise options, too. After six weeks of regular exercising you will really notice a difference. And don't

SPRING
The beginning of Spring is the ideal time to perform the one-month detox plan.

WINTER
Winter is not an ideal time to detox because your body needs plenty of nourishment to keep it fighting fit. However, if you are fit and well, you can follow a week of the month-long detox weekday plan (ie eating plenty of healthy wholefood).

forget to stretch – before and after exercising, or just for the sheer joy of it.

- Continue to practise the deep breathing until it becomes as natural as your "normal" breathing. Remind yourself of all the benefits.

- Keep an eye on your stress levels and find time for meditation, mindfulness, and/or relaxation exercises.

- Don't give up the skin brushing! You won't need to do it every time you bathe or shower but once a week is good.

- Give yourself a hydrotherapy treatment (see pp. 78-79) every so often. They are particularly useful if you have had a heavy night with too much rich food or alcohol (yes, we all have them!) or if you feel you are going down with a cold or flu.

- You may like to continue your journal, recording your dreams, your thoughts, and feelings. Equally, painting might become a part of your life. You may find these lead you naturally into seeking out some kind of psychotherapy or body therapy – if so, follow your natural instincts for this deep clearing.

SUMMER

This is the perfect time to have a week-long detox using plenty of fresh juices, fruits, and raw vegetables. Add in brown rice, chicken, fish, and lentils if you feel hungry or weak. You may also like to experiment with a short fast (see p. 102).

AUTUMN

Practise the weekend detox, making sure you use warm, cooked fruits and vegetables rather than raw and cold. Add warming spices.

THE DETOX YEAR

In addition to all the above, you can schedule various levels of more formal detox throughout the year (left).

TURNING YOUR HOME INTO A CHEMICAL-FREE SANCTUARY

There is one final aspect of your life you need to address
if you want to maintain your long-term detox. It is not
enough just to detox our bodies on the inside – we have
to take into account the world outside.

We all know about the pollution that surrounds us in
the outdoor environment – unfortunately, there is little we
can do about it on a personal level. However, we can take
charge of our homes and the products we bring into them.
There are a host of hidden toxins in the very fabric of our
homes and in the everyday products we use without a
second thought. Look back at the suggestions in Chapter
One for lessening the toxic overload in your home. If you
haven't already followed those guidelines, make an effort
to do so now. Now let's look a little more closely at how
you can help detox your entire lifestyle.

CHECK YOUR MEDICINE CABINET

The average household will have a whole array of over the
counter (OTC) medications around the home: a bottle or
two of pain-killers; cold and flu remedies; skin ointments
and lotions; treatments for corns and warts; mouth-
washes, antacids; cough syrups and sweets. However, as
with food additives, some of the active ingredients in OTC
preparations can cause allergic reactions. Others contain
drugs which may have unpleasant side effects.

The answer is to treat OTC preparations with huge
respect and caution: they are powerful drugs. If you can,
avoid using them: the great majority of minor ailments,
colds, and coughs will get better of their own accord.
In fact, suppressing symptoms with, for example, cold
remedies, can sometimes make the illness last longer.
If you have a serious problem, see your doctor. And you
should always consult your physician before self-treatment
if you are taking any prescription medications or other
OTC preparations. Then again, you could always start to
investigate the wide world of complementary healthcare,
which offers a huge array of safe natural alternatives for
OTC medications. Herbalism, nutritional therapy, and
homeopathy in particular offer very effective alternatives
to many common remedies. If you suffer from chronic

THE NATURAL FIRST AID KIT

Fennel tea bags: useful for digestive problems, from indigestion to flatulence.

Ginger powder: helps ease nausea and sickness (including morning sickness), travel sickness.

Aloe vera gel: use for acne, bites and stings, burns, cuts, sunburn, itchiness, and wounds.

Arnica ointment: use for back pain, bruises, joint pain, muscle aches and sprains, to reduce pain and swelling. **caution:** *not to be used on open wounds or broken skin. Some skins are sensitive to it so apply carefully when using for the first time.*

*Echinacea tincture **or tablets**: useful for all infections, echinacea raises the body's resistance to infection and speeds recovery. Use for colds, flu, digestive infections, earache, mouth ulcers, sore throats, thrush, cuts and grazes, catarrh and sinus problems, asthma, and warts. Echinacea can safely be taken with antibiotics and helps to reduce their side effects.*

*Garlic **capsules or tablets**: a natural antibiotic, use garlic for all kinds of infections (as for echinacea). It is particularly useful for infections in the nose, throat, and chest.*

*Lavender **essential oil**: a gentle pain reliever, lavender helps headaches and migraine (rub a few drops into the temples). Put 5 drops in a bath to encourage a good night's sleep.* **note:** *do not take internally.*

*Calendula ointment, **tincture, and tea**: use when the skin is red, sore and angry – it is healing and anti-inflammatory. Put the tincture on cuts and grazes (diluted in four parts of water for children); use the ointment for athlete's foot and for itchy skin in children. Taken internally, marigold tea eases heartburn, acidity, and upset digestion.*

Aconite 6x: homeopathic remedy for colds that come on suddenly; and for dry, harsh coughs that come on without warning.

Nux vomica 6x: homeopathic remedy for headache and nausea caused by over-indulgence of food or drink.

Arsen. Alb. 6x: very useful homeopathic remedy in cases of sickness from suspected bad food.

*Slippery elm powder **or tablets**: can produce dramatic results in acid indigestion, gastritis, diarrhea, constipation, bronchitis, and coughs. You can even plug a loose filling with slippery elm while a poultice of slippery elm and marigold tincture will draw out splinters and the pus from boils.*

*Tea tree **essential oil**: a potent yet gentle antiseptic, apply neat to small areas such as acne spots or around a nail. Use diluted (10 drops to 5ml/0.2fl.oz of almond oil or marigold ointment) on larger areas.* **caution:** *do not apply the oil neat on young children. Keep away from the eyes as even diluted it can sting.*

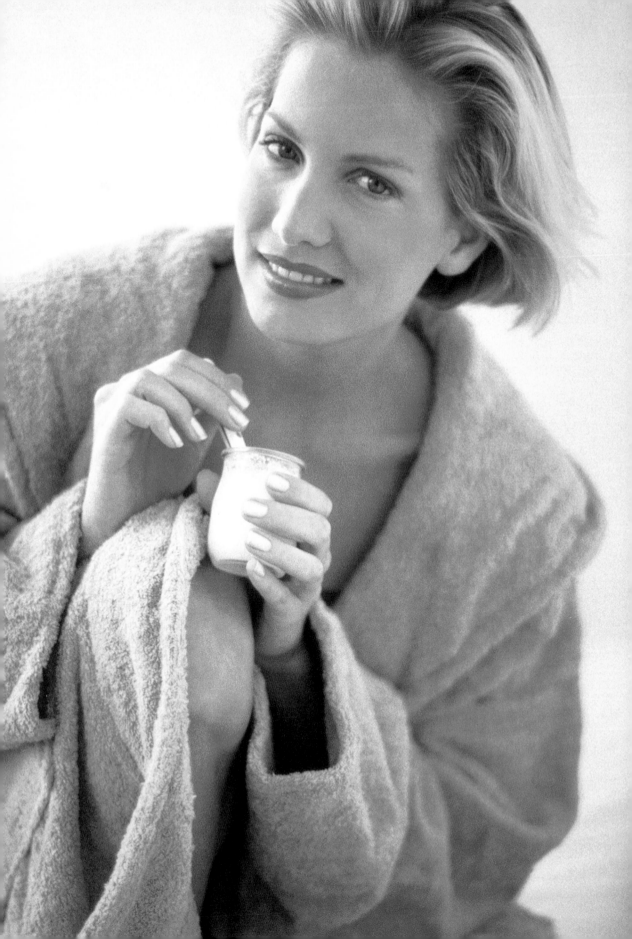

complaints such as arthritis, eczema, asthma, or digestive problems, consider a well-qualified complementary therapist, such as a nutritional therapist, herbalist, homeopath, or acupuncturist. Many people have found that, with simple changes to their diet, exercise, and lifestyle they can give up even prescription drugs.

SAFEGUARDING YOUR HEALTH – WHAT YOU CAN DO

Before you take any drug, find out as much about it as possible. Every drug marketed has a data sheet which gives a complete profile, listing when it should and shouldn't be taken, and also its side effects. They can be found in one of the following: the Data Sheet Compendium, the US Physicians Desk Reference, the Canadian Compendium of Pharmaceuticals & Specialities, the Cumulated Index Medicus, and MIMS (check with your local reference library or visit a large medical bookshop). Some libraries also have Medline, a computerized version of the Cumulated Index Medicus.

Never panic and come straight off drugs. Visit your doctor if you are concerned and go through all the medications you take, both prescription and OTC. Ask about any potential clashes; ask about alternatives.

If you are prescribed a drug by your doctor always tell him or her about any OTC preparations you are taking or sometimes take.

Don't automatically reach for a pill when you have a minor problem. Try gentle, natural alternatives. A great many complaints can be eliminated with correct diet and uncovering any food or chemical allergies.

BEAUTY PRODUCTS AND COSMETICS

The beauty business is a huge international industry, founded on our desperate desire to stay looking young and beautiful. But the side effects of many products can be less than glamorous. A large number of people find they are allergic to the common ingredients in cosmetics and beauty products, even simple products like shampoo and soap, after-shave, and antiperspirant. Even tiny amounts of these ingredients might cause eczema and acne, asthma and dermatitis. Perfumes are the most likely suspects

NATURAL BEAUTY ALTERNATIVES

If you make your own beauty preparations you can control precisely what goes into them. Some are just as effective – and much cheaper – than bought products. Try the following:

*Rosewater makes a superb **mild toner**, suitable for most skins.*

__Natural hair colours__ will rarely be as bright as chemicals but can give a wonderful sheen and lustre. Try strong tea as a final rinse to darken grey hair. Walnuts can darken and enhance hair colour (add 100g/4oz chopped walnuts to 600ml (1pt) of boiling water, strain, apply to the hair, and leave for 15 to 20 minutes). Elderberries will add a mahogany colour to dark hair; chamomile will bring out blonde hints in fair hair – simmer a large handful for 20 minutes in water, strain, and use as a herbal rinse. Henna is the age-old way to turn hair a rich bright red.

*Make your own **moisturizer** by melting 5g (0.18oz) of yellow beeswax and 40ml/1.6fl.oz of almond oil in a bain marie (a basin suspended over a pan of simmering water). Heat 10ml (0.4fl.oz) of rosewater in another basin until it is warm. Add the warm water to the oil and wax, drop by drop, beating with a whisk. Add 1 teaspoon of walnut oil. Bottle in sterilized glass pots, cover, and keep in the refrigerator. If you are prone to allergic reactions, patch test yourself for beeswax and almond oil. If you are not allergic to them you could add two drops of essential oil: choose lavender for oily, normal, or sensitive skin; rose for dry or aging skin.*

*You can make a simple **cleanser** by whisking one tablespoon of buttermilk with one tablespoon of lemon juice. Apply with cotton wool and rinse well with tepid water.*

*Eggs make a wonderful **hair conditioner** – simply beat four eggs and add a measure of rum. Massage into the scalp, followed by a rinse of cold water – don't use hot water, it would make the egg sticky.*

__Freckles__ look attractive and healthy but if you hate them try this instead of commercial products: pound two tablespoons of dried rosehips to a powder and mix to a paste with two teaspoons of cucumber juice. Apply as a mask for 15 minutes.

*There are several alternatives to **sunburn creams**: use slices of cucumber or cucumber juice; strong cold tea; neat cider vinegar; live plain yogurt (messy but effective); the juice of house-leek.*

*Make a natural **lip salve** using 30g/1oz of beeswax, 30ml/1.2fl.oz each of apricot and wheatgerm oil. Melt them all together in a bain marie and then take off the heat and continue stirring while the mixture cools. You could add three drops of lavender oil when the mixture is lukewarm. Test all ingredients for sensitivity.*

*A very simple and effective **toothpaste** can be made simply by mixing salt and bicarbonate of soda in equal parts.*

__Eye tonic:__ If your eyes are sore and puffy, cut two slices of raw potato and place them over your closed eyes. Lie down quietly and relax like this for 15 to 20 minutes. Teabags are also useful. Allow two used teabags to cool and then place over your eyelids for ten minutes. They will help reduce puffiness and dark circles.

followed by preservatives. All cosmetics and toiletries, even those which are "natural", are preserved. Some contain preservatives that are natural (such as grapefruit seed extract, tea tree oil, and some other essential oils) but they do not work alone, and usually need at least one of the synthetic preservatives for the product to be effective. Those who are prone to allergies often turn to "hypoallergenic" products but unfortunately there is no such thing as an entirely non-allergenic product: there is always someone who is allergic to something. Hypoallergenic products usually leave out around 60 known allergenics yet many more can, and do, cause allergic reactions.

SAFEGUARDING YOUR SKIN

There are simple ways to protect your skin – and your health. Follow these guidelines.

▪ Find out what is in the products you buy on a regular basis. If you write to the manufacturer of your favourite products they should provide you with a list of the ingredients. If they are unwilling to give out such information it's probably time for a change.

▪ Read all labels carefully and follow instructions exactly – particularly if using hair dyes, perms, freckle creams, skin packs, depilatories, and antiperspirants.

▪ If in any doubt about a product, try a patch test. Apply a small amount on the inside of your forearm and leave for 24 hours. If you see any adverse effects such as redness, itching, or blistering, do not use the product.

▪ If you have any adverse reaction to a cosmetic – stinging, itching, burning, etc. – stop using it. If you are not sure which product causes the problem, stop the use of all cosmetics – use only unscented soap on your skin and hair. Remove all nail polish. After a couple of weeks, re-introduce products one at a time.

▪ Do not breathe in products. Use compact powder rather than loose. Apply nail polish carefully, making sure it doesn't splash onto surrounding skin.

▪ Keep all cosmetics and beauty products well out of the reach of children. Many are highly toxic if ingested or inhaled.

- Avoid aerosol products which can lead to inhalation of chemicals – there are now many alternatives.
- Never keep cosmetics or beauty products beyond their use-by date: they can become rancid and cause infections, pimples, and acne.
- Choose alternatives to deodorants and antiperspirants. Natural "stone" products and other alternatives are available from health stores.
- Try to avoid synthetic hair colouring products. Choose natural products such as henna or chamomile. If you must colour, try "streaking" hair which reduces chemical exposure. Wear gloves when applying; don't leave the dye on your head any longer than necessary; rinse your scalp thoroughly after use. Never mix together different hair dye products. Be sure to do a patch test for allergic reactions before applying.
- Avoid products which are brightly coloured or strongly perfumed – they are more likely to cause allergies and adverse reactions.
- Try sugaring instead of depilatory creams.
- Get back to basics as much as possible. Many naturopaths say we should concentrate on gently cleansing the skin above all. Then put moisturizer on a damp skin. We really don't need all these liposomes, AHAs, biogenics, and so on.
- Stay out of the sun, wear a hat and protective clothing, and cultivate the "pale and interesting" look. Make sure children stay covered.
- Try natural face-savers: drink at least four glasses of still purified water a day. Eat a balanced low-fat diet with plenty of organic fruit and vegetables. Cut out smoking and cut down on alcohol (if you can't manage this, then take a supplement with B vitamins, vitamin C, and magnesium to counteract the effects on your skin). Make sure you get enough sleep and relaxation.
- Don't automatically trust labels promising "natural" or "herbal" – always check the label. Naturopaths give a simple rule of thumb: if the ingredient is too long to say, it's too chemical to go on your face.

THE HEALING HOME

Finally, remember that your home is your sanctuary from the world, a place in which you should feel safe, relaxed, and secure. So don't aim just to make it non-toxic and environmentally friendly. Aspire to a home with a heart, one which actively makes you feel better – healthier, happier, and more serene.

▪ Make a commitment to turning your home into a chemical-free sanctuary. Whenever you decorate or buy new furnishings, make sure they are toxin-free, and as natural as possible. Find out more from books like *The New Natural House Book* by David Pearson (see p. 124). There are now a host of companies producing non-toxic paints, varnishes, fabrics, and building materials. And discover the joy of reclaimed wood for furniture and flooring.

▪ Indulge all your senses – your home shouldn't just look good, it should feel good, smell good, sound good, and even taste good! Think about interesting textures underfoot; let beautiful aromatherapy scents waft through your home (instead of chemical air fresheners); and enjoy your favourite music. Keep vases full of colourful and fragrant flowers. Turn bowls into cornucopias of luscious fruit. Plant tubs with delightful bulbs. Place interesting stones all over your home.

▪ Investigate feng shui in greater depth and try to understand the way the energy flows in your home. Remember your home is more than a base for your body; it is a shelter for your spirit, too. Does your home inspire you? Make space for beautiful things: crafts lovingly made by hand; pictures, sculptures, or images which make your spirit soar.

▪ Try to have a space which you can call your own within your home. It needn't be a whole room, just a corner or a chair would do. We all need time alone, with our thoughts, so our minds can gently detox away from the hurly-burly of everyday life.

Resources

CHAPTER ONE

Dowsing

The Geo Group,
PO Box 602,
Medina, WA 98039
chuckp@geo.org.
Offer a geopathic survey
service. Website :
http://www.geo.org

CHAPTER TWO

Chi kung

The International Chi
Kung/Qi Gong Directory,
2730 29th Street,
Boulder, CO 80301
(303) 442-3131
or contact James
MacRitchie, founding
president of the group,
P. O. Box 19708,
Boulder, CO 80308

Yoga

International Association of
Yoga Therapists,
20 Sunnyside Avenue,
Suite A243,
Mill Valley, CA 94941
(415) 332-2478
(800) 858-9462

Integral Yoga Teachers'
Association,
Route 1 Box 1720,
Buckingham, VA 23921
www.moonstar.com/~yoga
Also try www.yogacite.com
and www.yogajournal.com
as good sources of
information about teachers.

Tai chi

Look in your health/sports
center for local classes. Or
contact: Alexander Krych,
c/o Belvidere Post Office,
Belvidere, NJ 07823-2018
(908) 475-1619
74640.2154@compuserve.
com

Biodanza

Denise Melo,
1104 Willingham Way,
Moore, OK 73160
(405) 794-0500

CHAPTER THREE

Feng shui

William Spear,
24 Village Green Drive,
Litchfield, CT 06759
(860) 567-8801
fengshuime@aol.com

Counseling

American Counseling
Association,
5999 Stevenson Avenue,
Alexandria, VA 22304
(703) 823-9800

Bach flower remedies

Nelson Bach USA Ltd.,
100 Research Drive,
Wilmington, MA 01887
(978) 988-3833

Flower essence services

FES
P. O. Box 1769,
Nevada City, CA 95959

(916) 265-9163
FES Quintessentials line of
North American flower
essences.

Flower Essence Society
P. O. Box 459
Nevada City, CA 95959
(916) 265-9163

Meditation

Check your health center
for classes. TM – Maharishi
University of Management
Fairfield, IA 52557 (515)
472-1134. TM has teachers
all over the US.

CHAPTER FOUR

Naturopathy

American Association of
Naturopathic Physicians,
601 Valley Street # 105,
Seattle, WA 98105
(206) 298-0126
and referrals – (206) 298-
0125

American Naturopathic
Medical Association,
P. O. Box 96273,
Las Vegas, NV 89193
(702) 897-7053

Bastyr University of
Natural Health Sciences
14500 Juanita Drive NE,
Bothell, WA 98011
(425) 823-1300

National Institute of
Nutritional Education,
1010 S. Joliet Street 107,
Aurora, CO 80012
(303) 340-2054

Aromatherapy
American Aromatherapy
Association,
P. O. Box 3609,
Culver City, CA 90231

Aromatherapy Institute of
Research,
P. O. Box 2354,
Fair Oaks, CA 95628
(916) 965-7546

Massage
American Massage Therapy
Association,
820 Davis Street, Suite 100,
Evanston, IL 60201-4444
(847) 864-0123

Associated Bodywork and
Massage Professionals,
28677 Buffalo Park Road,
Evergreen, CO 80439-7347
(303) 674-8478

The Feldenkrais Guild,
P. O. Box 489,
Albany, OR 97321
(541) 926-0981

Reiki Alliance,
P. O. Box 41,
Cataldo, ID 83810
(208) 682-3535

Trager Institute,
21 Locust Avenue,
Mill Valley, CA 94941
(415) 388-2688

MANAGING LONG-TERM DETOX
Beauty products
Some companies use only
natural ingredients – look
out for Jurlique, Kiehls,
and Aveda. Your health
store should also have
chemical-free products.

Other helpful organizations
After detoxing, you may
want to investigate natural
methods of healing further.
My first two books,
Supertherapies and *The
Natural Year* (both
Bantam), outline a host of
healing therapies and give
suggestions for putting
your body back into
balance. For further
information, try these
organizations:

Arica Institute, Inc.,
145 Palisade Street,
Suite 401,
Dobbs Ferry, NY 10522
(914) 674-4091

Homeopathy
Homeopathic Academy of
Naturopathic Physicians,
P. O. Box 69565,
Portland, OR 97201
(503) 761-3298

International Foundation
for Homeopathy,
2366 Eastlake Ave. E, 329
Seattle, WA 98102
(425) 776-4147

The National Center for
Homeopathy,
801 N. Fairfax, Suite 306,
Alexandria, VA 22314
(703) 548-7790

Medical herbalism
American Botanical
Council,
P. O. Box 201660,
Austin, TX 78720
(512) 331-8868

American Herbalists Guild,
P. O. Box 1683,
Sequel, CA 95973
(408) 484-2441

*Traditional Chinese
medicine/acupuncture*
American Association of
Oriental Medicine,
433 Front Street,
Catasauqua, PA 18032
(610) 266-1433

Ayurveda
Ayurvedic Institute,
11311 Menaud NE,
Suite A,
Albuquerque, NM 87112
(505) 291-9698

Useful reading

GENERAL DETOXING

A short, simple book is *Detox Yourself* by Jane Scrivner (Piatkus). *You are What you Eat* by Kirsten Hartvig and Dr Nic Rowley (Piatkus) is a good guide to naturopathic principles and includes some detoxing. For deeper insights read *Detoxification & Healing* by Dr Sidney MacDonald Baker (Keats Publishing). My book *The Natural Year* (Bantam) gives guidelines for eating healthily throughout the year with seasonal detox programs. It also gives ideas on exercise and the kinds of issues you might address while detoxing.

DETOXING THE HOME

By far the best book available is *The New Natural House Book* by David Pearson (Simon & Schuster, 1998), which tells you all you need to know to make your home a safe haven. *H is for ecoHome* by Anna Kruger (Avon, 1992) is an A-Z guide to making your house healthy and toxin free. *Clean House, Clean Planet* by Karen Logan (Pocket Books, 1997) is a brilliant guide to keeping your home clean without using toxic materials. *Folk Wisdom for a Natural Home* by Beverly Pagram (Trafalgar, 1997) is inspirational and beautiful. It really makes you want to start cleaning! *C is for Chemicals* by Michael Birkin and Brian Price (Green Print) is a classic on the dangers of chemicals in everyday household products – it also offers safe alternatives. *Silent Spring* by Rachel Carson (Houghton Mifflin, 1994) argues against the indiscriminate use of chemicals in society – first published in 1962, it is (sadly) still relevant and vital reading if you are concerned about your health and the environment.

FOOD AND NUTRITION

Secret Ingredients by Peter Cox and Peggy Brusseau (Bantam) lists many chemicals and other "hidden" ingredients in food, over the counter remedies, and home products. Terrifying but illuminating. *The Nutritional Health Bible* by Linda Lazarides (Thorsons) is excellent on nutritional therapy and supplementation.
Also useful when following a long-term detox plan are: *A Diet for All Seasons* by Elson M Haas MD (Celestial Arts, 1995)
The Ayurvedic Cookbook by Amadea Morningstar with Urmila Desai (Lotus Light, 1990)
Gluten-Free Cookery by Peter Thomson (Trafalgar, 1996)
Moosewood Restaurant Low-Fat Favorites by the Moosewood Collective (Crown Publishing Group, 1997)
Eat More, Weigh Less by Dean Ornish MD (Harper San Francisco, 1997). Don't be put off by the title – it has good low-fat, allergen-free recipes.

BREATHING

Breathing into Life by Bija Bennett (Harper San Francisco) is a lovely little book, full of practical advice and inspirational wisdom.
Two good introductory books on yoga are: *Yoga for Common Ailments* by Drs R Nagarathna, Nagendra, and Monro (Simon & Schuster, 1991) and *Yoga for Long Life* by Stella Weller (Thorsons).

CHI KUNG

The Way of Qigong by Kenneth S Cohen (Bantam) and *The Art of Chi Kung* by Wong Kiew Kit (Element, 1996) are well worth reading.

REBOUNDING

Starbound by Michele Wilburn (Orion) gives you all you need for the perfect rebounding workout.

TAI CHI

I think it is impossible to learn tai chi accurately from a book. But if you cannot find a class and are keen to start, *The Tai Chi Manual* by Robert Parry (Piatkus) is probably the clearest guide.

PILATES

Body Control, The Pilates Way by Lynne Robinson and Gordon Thomson (Trans-Atlantic Publications, 1997) is a great way to get started in your own home.

PSYCHONEUROIMMUNOLOGY

PNI by Dr Elliott S Dacher (Marlowe, 1994) explains mind-body medicine in some detail and gives practical exercises for helping your entire being work in harmony.

FENG SHUI

My all-time favorite feng shui book is *Interior Design with Feng Shui* by Sarah Rossbach (Rider), which is clear and authoritative.
My favorite from the new batch is *Feng Shui for your Home* by Sarah Shurety (Viking Penguin, 1991). *The Feng Shui House Book* by Gina Lazenby (Conran) is also beautiful and inspirational.
Karen Kingston's book *Creating Sacred Space with Feng Shui* (Broadway Books, 1997) is excellent on decluttering your home.
My book *Spirit of the Home* (Thorsons) introduces feng shui and space cleansing and looks at ways to make your home a healing sanctuary.

TIME MANAGEMENT

The following are useful: *Effective Time Management* by John Adair (Pan). *Better Time Management* by Jacqueline Atkinson (Thorsons). *Making Time Work For You* by Marek Gitlin (Sheldon).

STRESS RELIEF

Body Wisdom by Amiyo Ruhnke and Anando Wurzburger (Charles E.

Tuttle, 1996) is one of my favorite books – it gives easy yet powerful exercises and self-massage techniques for people on the go. A "must-have" if you work in an office.

The Complete Guide to Reducing Stress by Christine Wildwood (London Bridge, 1997) is a good guide to various methods of relaxation. *Stress Management* by Vera Pfeiffer (Thorsons) is sensible, straightforward, and very useful. *Stopping* by David Kundtz offers ways to bring back meaning to life. Highly recommended. *Downshifting* by Andy Bull (Thorsons) could simplify your lifestyle to cut down on stress.

MEDITATION AND MINDFULNESS

The 3 Minute Meditator by David Harp with Nina Feldman (New Harbinger Publications, 1996) is perfect for meditation plus it offers 30 simple relaxation techniques. *Wherever You Go There You Are: Mindfulness Meditation for Everyday Life* by Jon Kabat-Zinn (Hyperion) is the classic on mindfulness techniques. *Finding the Stillness Within in a Busy World* by Sue Vaughan (National Book Network, 1995) is a helpful book on meditation.

TOXIC EMOTIONS

The Worrywort's Companion by Dr Beverly Potter (Wildcat Canyon Press) is a lovely little book which gives 21 ways to beat worrying. *The Dance of Anger* by Harriet G Lerner (HarperCollins, 1989) is wise, insightful, and practical on anger management. *The Nice Factor Book* by Robin Chandler and Jo Ellen Grzyb (Simon & Schuster) is ideal for addressing your own needs if you are too nice for your own good. *The Assertive Woman* by Stanlee Phelps and Nancy Austin (Impact) is a classic in assertiveness training.

The 60-Second Shrink by Arnold A Lazarus and Clifford N Lazarus (Impact) is packed with useful strategies for dealing with difficult situations and toxic emotions.

FLOWER REMEDIES

The best all-round guide is *The Encyclopaedia of Flower Remedies* by Clare G Harvey and Amanda Cochrane (Thorsons, 1995). *The Complete Floral Healer* by Anne McIntyre (Henry Holt, 1996) is also very informative (it also covers herbs, aromatherapy, and homeopathy). *Keys to the Soul* by Mechthild Scheffer (C W Daniel) is a workbook for emotional and spiritual growth.

HYDROTHERAPY

The Complete Book of Water Healing by Dian Dincin Buchman (Instant Improvement, 1995) is ideal if you want to go further with water – it gives 500 ways to use water therapeutically! I also like *Water Magic* by Mary Muryn (Simon & Schuster, 1995), which gives lovely ideas for healing and magical baths but no naturopathic or detox techniques.

FOOD ALLERGIES & ELIMINATION DIETS

The Elimination Diet Cookbook and *The Rotation Diet Cookbook* (both by Element, 1997) by Jill Carter and Alison Edwards are both very clear and offer a more detailed approach to elimination than I am able to give in this book. *Natural Way Allergies* by Moira Crawford (Element, 1998) is a short, straightforward, but informative introduction.

AROMATHERAPY

The Fragrant Pharmacy by Valerie Ann Worwood (Bantam), Tricia Davies' *A-Z of Aromatherapy* (C W Daniels), and *The Encyclopedia of Aromatherapy* by Christine

Wildwood (Inner Traditions International).

MASSAGE

The Complete Illustrated Guide to Massage by Stewart Mitchell (Element, 1997) gives clear instructions on home massage.

ALTERNATIVE REMEDIES

My book *Supertherapies* (Bantam) gives the lowdown on over 40 types of holistic health treatments. *What's the Alternative?* by Hazel Courteney and Dr John Briffa (Boxtree) lists alternatives for over 150 common conditions. *The New Natural Family Doctor* edited by Dr Andrew Stanway (North Atlantic Books, 1996) and *The Complete Family Guide to Natural Home Remedies* (Element) are good reference guides. For advice on homeopathy I turn to *The Family Guide to Homeopathy* by Dr Andrew Lockie and Dr Nicola Geddes (Simon & Schuster, 1993)

COSMETICS/NATURAL BEAUTY

A Consumer's Dictionary of Cosmetic Ingredients by Ruth Winter (Crown Publishing Group, 1994) is an exhaustive list of what goes into beauty products and what they can do to you. *What's in Your Cosmetics* by Aubrey Hampton (Odonian, 1995) is not as encyclopedic but has a useful section on natural alternatives. My favorite natural beauty book is *The New Beauty* by Michelle Dominique Leigh (Kodansha, 1995) – a wonderful guide to East-West beauty techniques using natural methods. *Absolute Beauty* by Pratima Raichur (Bantam) comes a close second – an inspirational guide to beauty using Ayurvedic principles.

Books from Tuttle Publishing and Journey Editions

Breathing
Beginning Yoga by Dr. Vijayendra Pratap
(Charles E. Tuttle Co., Inc., 1997)

Chi Kung
*Ch'i the Power Within: Chi Kung Breathing Exercises for Health,
Relaxation and Energy* (Charles E. Tuttle Co., Inc., 1996)

Feng Shui
The Feng Shui Workbook by Wu Xing (Charles E. Tuttle Co., Inc., 1998)
guides you room-by-room through your home to improve its feng shui.

Healing Design: A Book of Feng Shui (Journey Editions, 1998)
by Hope Gerecht, an interior designer, gives you ways of improving the
flow of chi in your home.

Meditation and Mindfulness
The Everyday Meditator by Osho (Charles E. Tuttle Co., Inc., 1993)
is filled with simple techniques to help you incorporate meditation
into your everyday life.

The Meditation Kit by Charla Devereux (Journey Editions, 1997)
is a comprehensive resource for beginning meditators and includes practical
instructions on breathing techniques, the uses of mandalas, and visualization.

Meditation for Absolutely Everyone by Subagh Singh Khalsa
(Charles E. Tuttle Co., Inc., 1994) gives straightforward guidance on meditation.

Toxic Emotions
The Stress Management Kit by Alix Needham (Journey Editions, 1996)
offers a system to help you recognize, understand, and reduce stress
in your daily life.

Aromatherapy
The Aromatherapy Kit by Charla Devereux (Charles E. Tuttle Co., Inc., 1993)

Cosmetics/Natural Beauty
The Natural Beauty Kit by Joanna Sheen (Journey Editions, 1997)
features recipes for making your own natural beauty products.

Index

ACKNOWLEDGMENTS

In particular I would like to thank
Antony Haynes of The Nutrition
Clinic and Sue Weston. Antony
checked the detox programs and
made valuable suggestions. Sue
advised on the chi kung and toxic
emotions sections of the book.

Also a profound thank-you to the
very many therapists and
practitioners whose wisdom I have
plundered over the years. I must
acknowledge Fiona Arrigo whose
superb Stop the World program
introduced me to detoxing; also
Nicola Griffin, Lynne Crawford and
the staff of Tyringham Hall
Naturopathic Clinic.

My sincere thanks go to all the
Gaia team – in particular Pip
Morgan and Phil Gamble who
worked so hard on this project. And
to Eleanor Lines and Lyn Hemming
who got the ball rolling.

As always, many "gratitude
moments" to Judy Chilcote, the best
agent and friend a writer could have.